# Animal Productivity and Nutritional Security

## THE EDITORS

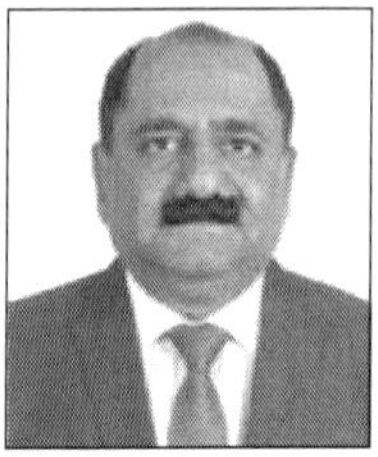

**Dr. Sunil Nayak**, presently working as Director Extension education, Nanaji Deshmukh Veterinary Science University, Jabalpur (M.P.). Dr. Nayak was born on 27th June, 1965 in Madhya Pradesh. He joined as Assistant Professor in Department of Animal Nutrition, College of Veterinary Science and A.H., N.D.V.S.U., Jabalpur (M.P.) in the year 1995. He had 23 years of experience in Teaching, Research and Extension. He had guided many M.V.Sc. and 02 Ph.D. students as major advisor & handled 2 research projects as PI. He had published many lead articles & more than 100 research papers in the Journals of National & International repute. Major research achievements of Dr. Nayak include contributions in Poultry Nutrition. He is author of 1 book, many technical bulletins, annual reports, 8 manuals, more than 120 popular articles, extension booklets, folder and leaflets. He is life member of 10 different National & International Scientific Societies. On account of his scientific recognition and regards, he had been nominated as Vice President of Animal Nutrition Association of India and Executive Member Animal Nutrition Society of India.

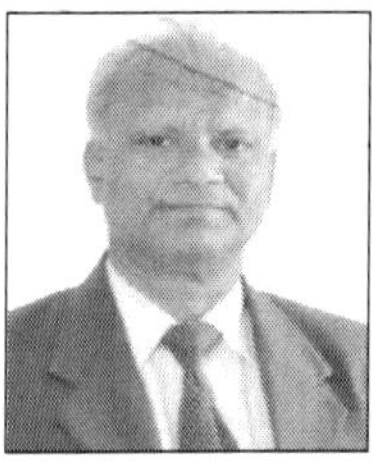

**Dr. Ramesh Pratap Singh Baghel**, presently Dean Faculty of Veterinary Science at Nanaji Deshmukh Veterinary Science University, Jabalpur (M.P.). He was born on 15th September 1956 at Rampur Baghelan in Satna district of Madhya Pradesh. He was awarded Bachelor's degree in Veterinary Science and Animal Husbandry and Master's in Animal Nutrition from J.N.K.V.V., Jabalpur and received University Gold Medals in Bachelors and Post Graduate Degree programmes. He completed his Ph.D. from C.C. Haryana Agri. Univ. Hisar, Haryana in 1987 and was awarded with Dr. S.K.Ranjhan Best Ph.D. Thesis award. During his service period, he has guided 2 Ph.D., 25 M.V.Sc. and 25 M.Phil students as major advisor. He has vast experience of work in the livestock production (dairy, poultry, goat and pig laboratory animals) and extension. He published more than 250 research articles in the Journals of National and International repute. He has published books and bulletins in Hindi as well as English. He has also handled 2 research projects of ICAR as PI and two as Co-PI. He is also the "Fellow" National Academy of Veterinary Sciences, India. He is life member of eight different national scientific societies.

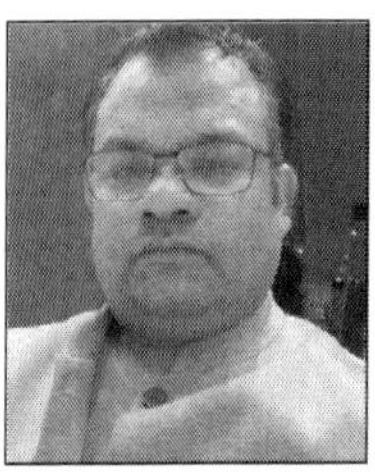

**Dr. Ankur Khare**, presently working as an assistant professor in the Department of Animal Nutrition, CoVSc & A.H. Jabalpur (M.P.). He was born on 29th July, 1981 in Bhopal, M.P. He joined as Assistant Professor in Department of Animal Nutrition, College of Veterinary Science and A.H., N.D.V.S.U., Jabalpur (M.P.) in the year 2015. He had work as a JRF and SRF under AICRP project of Indian Council of Agriculture Research for 8 years. He had published 42 research papers in National & International Journals. He is author of 1 book, 02 technical bulletins, 08 annual reports, 03 manuals, and 53 popular articles. He is life member of 07 different National Societies. He is also a Fellow member of society of life sciences. Due to his exemplary work in livestock Nutrition under AICRP, Society of life science also awarded him with "Extra Ordinary Research Achievements" in the field of livestock nutrition.

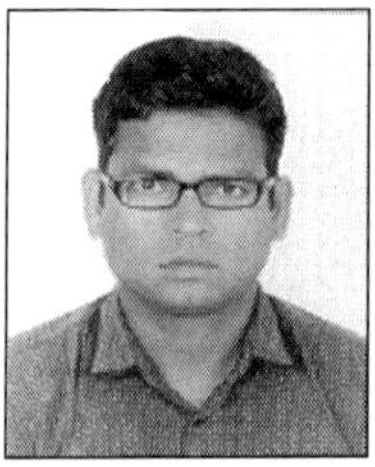

**Dr. Ravi Prakash Pal** (Teaching Associate) Department of Animal Nutrition, Co.V.Sc. & A.H., Jabalpur (M.P.). He was born on 8th January 1987 in Jaunpur, Uttar Pradesh. He has completed his graduation (BVSc & AH) from CoVSc & AH, Jabalpur (M.P.) and continued his postgraduate and doctorate degree from NDRI, Karnal. He had published 21 research papers in National and International journals. He is author of 03 manual, 07 book chapter, 04 lead article and 25 popular articles. He is also a life member of 07 different professional societies. He is awarded with fellowship during M.V.Sc. and Ph.D. degree. He is also awarded with young scientist award in conference of Association of Animal Scientist-2020.

# Animal Productivity and Nutritional Security

*— Editors —*

**Sunil Nayak**

**R.P.S. Baghel**

**Ankur Khare**

**Ravi Prakash Pal**

BIOTECH

2022

**BIOTECH BOOKS®**

concepts without unessential details. Through this format, my goal is to give students the tools and help to understand animal nutrition by focusing on some key topics and concepts.

I hope that the book will provide useful information on animal nutrition to students worldwide.

***Sunil Nayak***

***R.P.S. Baghel***

***Ankur Khare***

***Ravi Prakash Pal***

# Contents

Chapter 1

# Feed Resources: Availability, Challenges and Feed Security in India

*R.P.S. Baghel, Ankur Khare, S. Nayak and Pramod Sharma*

*Department of Animal Nutrition, College of Veterinary Science and Animal Husbandry, Nanaji Deshmukh Veterinary Science University, Jabalpur, Madhya Pradesh*

India has one of the largest livestock populations in the world, and one of its notable characteristics is that almost its entire feed requirement is met from crop residues and byproducts, grasses, weeds and tree leaves gathered from cultivated and uncultivated lands, and grazing on common lands and harvested fields. Land allocation to cultivation of green fodder crops is limited and has hardly ever exceeded 5 per cent of the gross cropped area (GoI, 2009). Hence, the supply of feed has always remained short of normative requirement (Ramachandra *et al.*, 2007), restricting realization of the true production potential of livestock. Birthal and Jha (2005) have found feed scarcity as the main limiting factor to improving livestock productivity.

## Present Status of Animal Feed Resources

The feed and livestock resources has been assessed based on the secondary data on crop production, land utilization pattern for the last three years and livestock census obtained from the Directorate of Economics and Statistics and Department of Animal Husbandry and Veterinary Sciences, Government of India.

Availability of feed resources in terms of dry matter through crop residues, concentrates and greens for the period 2010-2050 is presented in Table 1.2. Contrary to the belief that there has been a decline in the availability of feed resources, the data clearly shows that the overall dry matter availability from different sources has increased over the years from 341 million tonnes to 574 million tonnes. The increased availability of feed resources was chiefly due to the increase in the crop residues and to a limited extent by increase in the concentrates. Availability of greens was more or less remained static over the years.

## Crop Residues

These are generally defined as feedstuffs, which are bulky and contain more than 18 per cent fibre. Crop residues comprise straws and stovers obtained after harvesting the crops. Crop residues are the major feed resource for feeding of livestock across all states. The states of Maharashtra, Andhra Pradesh and Karnataka, which were considered as traditional states cultivating the coarse cereals to a considerable extent have shown a declining trend over the years probably due to the change in the shifting cultivation from coarse cereal crops to rice cultivation. This has resulted in less availability of coarse straws for feeding of animals in these states.

## Concentrates

Concentrates as feed ingredients are less bulky, contain less than 18 per cent fibre and are rich in energy-yielding nutrients. Concentrates comprise of cereal grains and their by-products, oilseeds and their products and animal products. The availability of concentrates (on DM basis) through oil cakes, bran, chuni and grains has increased from 16.82 million tons in 1980-81 to 49.71 million tonnes in 2011-12 (oil cakes 19.6, bran and chunni 16.38 and grains 13.73).

## Green Fodder

There has not been much improvement in the availability of green fodder over the years, which is a matter of concern. The dry matter availability through greens on all India basis, which was 147.46 MT in 1980-81 has increased to 168.66 MT in 2011- 12 (Table 1.2). Even though the area under the cultivated fodder crops has increased over the years due to the increase in gross cropped area the percentage of the area under fodder cultivation has almost remained stagnant at 4 per cent of the total cropped area in the country.

Non-conventional feed resources (NCFR) generally refer to all those feeds that have not been traditionally used for feeding livestock and are not commercially used in the production of livestock feeds.

## Quality/Characteristics of NCFR

According to reports (FAO, 1985), non-conventional feed resources like conventional feed resources have several characteristics worthy of note.

a) They are the end products of production processes and consumption that have not been used, recycled or salvaged.
b) They are mostly of organic origin and can be obtained either in a solid, slurry or liquid form.
c) The economic value of these non-conventional feed resources is usually less than the cost of their collection and transformation for use and consequently, they are discharged as wastes.
d) Feed crops which generate valuable NCFR are usually excellent sources of fermentable nutrient molecules such as cassava and sweet potato and this is an advantage to livestock especially ruminants due to their ability to utilize inorganic nitrogen and non-protein nitrogenous sources.
e) Fruit wastes such as banana rejects and pineapple pulp by comparison have sugars which are energetically beneficial.

## Constraints to the Uses of Non-conventional Feed Resources

Non-conventional feed resources are presently underutilized and there are several reasons.

a) Production is usually scattered, the quality produced is low.
b) Sometimes cost of collection can be unusually high, for example, rubber seeds.
c) Processing of NCFR is usually difficult and can be problematic in certain cases.
d) Lack of managerial and technical skills in the utilization of such feeds in situ.
e) Limitation in the end uses of the products produced.
f) The uncertainty about the marketability of the end products.

## Agro-industrial By-products

The increasing human demands for several food types such as vegetables, wine, fruit juices *etc.*, has led to a considerable decrease in available farming lands due to the increase in the cropping of these foods. Consequently, this leads to an increase in the availability of agro-industrial by-products (AIBPs) such as molasses, brewer's dried grains, palm oil cake, winery mash and so on, which are not fully utilized in livestock feeding. Most of these products are low in major nutrients and do not form properly balanced diets (Devendra, 1983). The difficulty of the use of these feed sources as fresh material for extended periods and the lack of efficient ways for their integration in feeding regimes may account for their under-utilization (Chadhokar, 1984).

## Challenges

### Huge Livestock Resources and their Low Productivity

Urbanization has brought a marked shift in feeding habits of people towards milk, meat and eggs with the consequential increase in demand of livestock products. Meat and milk consumption will grow at 2.8 and 3.3 per cent per annum, respectively, in developing countries like India. The human population in India is expected to reach over 1531.4 million and 30 per cent urban population is poised to increase by over 75 per cent by 2050. The demand for milk and meat will be around 400 and 14 million tonnes, respectively in the year 2050; whereas the production in 2011 was about 122 and 5 million tonnes respectively.

**Table 1.1. Projected Livestock Population Estimates***
**(million Adult Cattle Unit, ACU#)**

| *Year* | *Cattle* | *Buffalo* | *Sheep* | *Goat* | *Equine* | *Camel* | *Total* |
|---|---|---|---|---|---|---|---|
| 2010 | 127.3 | 88.88 | 4.66 | 9.03 | 0.75 | 0.49 | 231.1 |
| 2020 | 129.1 | 95.31 | 5.03 | 10.32 | 0.63 | 0.43 | 240.8 |
| 2030 | 133.6 | 106.8 | 5.39 | 11.18 | 0.54 | 0.29 | 257.9 |
| 2040 | 136.6 | 115.0 | 5.76 | 11.99 | 0.40 | 0.20 | 270.1 |
| 2050 | 139.6 | 127.1 | 6.13 | 13.19 | 0.29 | 0.12 | 286.5 |

* Estimates based on past Livestock censuses published by the Directorate of Economic and Statistics and Department of Animal Husbandry and Dairying.

\# Category-wise population data was multiplied with standard body weight to get total weight while conversion to ACU (1 ACU = 350 kg).

### Shortage of Forage and Feed Resources

Forage based economical feeding strategies are required to reduce the cost of quality livestock product as the feed alone constitutes 60-70 per cent of the milk production cost. Thus any attempt towards enhancing feed availability and economizing the feed cost would result in increased margin of profits to livestock owners also. There is tremendous pressure of livestock on available total feed and fodder, as land available for fodder production has been decreasing. At present, the country faces a net deficit of 35.6 per cent green fodder, 10.95 per cent dry crop residues and 44 per cent concentrate feed ingredients. Supply and demand scenario of forage and roughage and grazing resources are presented in Tables 1.2 and 1.3, respectively.

**Table 1.2. Demand and Supply Estimates* of Dry and Freen Forages (million tonnes)**

| *Year* | *Demand* | | *Supply* | | *Deficit* | | *Deficit as per cent* | |
|---|---|---|---|---|---|---|---|---|
| | *Dry* | *Green* | *Dry* | *Green* | *Dry* | *Green* | *Dry* | *Green* |
| 2010 | 508.9 | 816.8 | 453.2 | 525.5 | 55.72 | 291.3 | 10.95 | 35.66 |
| 2020 | 530.5 | 851.3 | 467.6 | 590.4 | 62.85 | 260.9 | 11.85 | 30.65 |
| 2030 | 568.1 | 911.6 | 500.0 | 687.4 | 68.07 | 224.2 | 11.98 | 24.59 |
| 2040 | 594.9 | 954.8 | 524.4 | 761.7 | 70.57 | 193.0 | 11.86 | 20.22 |
| 2050 | 631.0 | 1012.7 | 547.7 | 826.0 | 83.27 | 186.6 | 13.20 | 18.43 |

*Source*: IGFRI (2013)

*Assumptions: For calculation of demand of dry and green forages, concentrate feed's data were adopted from article 'India's livestock feed demand: Estimates and projections.Dikshit, A.K., and P.S. Birthal. 2010. Agricultural Economics Research Review, 23(1):15-28.

**Table 1.3. Grazing Resources in India**

| *Resources* | *Area (million ha)* | *Percentage* |
|---|---|---|
| Forests | 69.41 | 22.70 |
| Permanent pastures, grazing lands | 10.90 | 3.60 |
| Cultivable wasteland | 13.66 | 4.50 |
| Fallow land | 24.99 | 8.10 |
| Fallow land other than current fallows | 10.19 | 3.30 |
| Barren uncultivable wastelands | 19.26 | 6.30 |
| Total common property resources | 54.01 | 17.70 |

*Source*: IGFRI (2013)

## Gaps and Shortcomings

Focus on prioritized area of forage research with commensurate allocation of manpower and material resources have been a major drawback. More specific gaps and shortcomings related to forage production are as under; Higher priority was given to research on cultivated fodder crops as compared to rangeland research in terms of manpower and investments. Grassland/silvipasture research needs to incorporate aspects of soil moisture conservation and water harvesting which could have increased total biomass productivity manifold under rainfed situation. There is not much understanding of tree-pasture-livestock interactions in total productivity context.

## Conclusion

Changing agriculture production practices, globalization of economy, money oriented production system, decentralized/democratic form of government have its impact on livestock production system in the country, therefore following policies may be focused in future:

- Look for good indigenous milch breed of cattle particularly for semi-arid climates, upgrade these breeds through recent techniques as animal as animal husbandry is main activity in such area.
- Adopt intensive and well defined milestones to achieve growth in production of indigenous breeds in such areas.
- Adopt breeds/cross breeds in areas commensurate with productivity of area *i.e.* in case of high agriculture production area, crossbreds with high potentials will be able to compete with agriculture crops.
- There should be focused programme on regeration, promotion of silvi-pasture and wastelands, which will not only meet shortcoming of feed and fodders but will give equal access to poor and improve environment also.
- There is need to promote fodder crop production through improved agronomic practices and use of improved seed.
- Presently research is mainly conducted on cultivation of green fodder in irrigated areas but focus has to be given to dry land fodder or partially irrigated fodder crops.

## REFERENCES

GoI (2009). Year-wise Area under Crops - All India. Available at: http: //dacnet.nic. in/eands/LUS-2006-07/Summary/tb3.13.pdf.

Singh, P. and Mujumdar, A.B. (1992). Current status of feed and forage management of livestock in India. *Agriculture Situation in India*, **47**(5): 375-382.

Ramachandra, K.S., Taneja, V.K., Sampath, K.T., Anandan, S. and Angadi, U.B. (2007). Livestock Feed Resources in Different Agro-ecosystems of India: Availability, Requirement and their Management. National Institute of Animal Nutrition and Physiology, Bangalore.

Birthal, P.S. and Jha, A.K. (2005). Economic losses due to various constraints in dairy production in India. *Indian Journal of Animal Sciences*, **75**: 1476-1480.

Gadde, B., Bonnet, S., Menke, C. and Garivait, S. (2009). Air pollutant emissions from rice straw open field burning in India, Thailand and the Philippines. *Environmental Pollution*, **157**(5): 1554-1558.

FAO, (1985). FAO/APHCA Publication: Non-conventional feed resources in Asia and the pacific (2nd ed). *FAO regional office for Asia and the Pacific, Bangkok*, 1985.

Devendra, C (1983). Small farm systems combining crops and animals. *In; Proceedings of the 5th World Conference on Animal Production.* Vol.1, pp. 173-191.

Chadhokar, P.A. (1984). Non-conventional feed resources for livestock in soil and water conservation program. Community Forestry and Soil Conservation Development Department, Ministry of Agric. FAO. Adis-Ababa, Ethiopia.

IGFRI (2013). Vision 2050. Indian Grassland and Fodder Research Institute, pp.1-40.

## Chapter 2

# Feeding Strategies to Enhance Milk Productivity in the Rural Areas

*Sunil Nayak, R.P.S. Baghel, Ankur Khare and Shanu Singour*

*Department of Animal Nutrition,*
*College of Veterinary Science and Animal Husbandry,*
*Nanaji Deshmukh Veterinary Science University, Jabalpur, Madhya Pradesh*

Milk is an important component of diets for all humans as it is high in essential amino acids that are most likely to be deficient in diets based on vegetable protein. Although milk is a high-cost source of protein and fat relative to vegetable sources, it is readily saleable particularly in the more affluent urban areas of developing countries. Improving milk production is therefore an important tool for improving the quality of life particularly for rural people in developing countries.

In spite of achieving the highest milk production (165.4 million tonnes in 2016-17) in the world, the performance of our cattle has been extremely poor. The country has a bovine population of 300 million as per 19$^{th}$ Livestock census 2012 and out of 190 million cattle population, 20 per cent are exotic and crossbreds (39 million) and about 80 per cent belonging to indigenous and Non-descript breeds. While India accounts for more than 18 per cent of the world population, the normal Indian cow with the poor farmer barely gives 1 to 2 litres per day. Thus 80 per cent of the cow population gives only 20 per cent of cow milk.

To meet the current level of livestock production and its annual growth in population, the deficit in all components of fodder, dry crop residues and feed has to be met either from increasing productivity, utilizing untapped feed resources, increasing land area (may not possible due to human pressure for food crops) or through imports.

## Feed Resources Available to Livestock

Dairy animals in India and other tropical countries are fed mainly on by-products of various food crops, oil seeds and locally grown fodder. Due to population pressure the land for fodder production has dwindled alarmingly and the cereal crop residues like paddy straw, wheat straw, sorghum straw *etc.* have become the major source of feed for large sections of the ruminant population. The available resources are essentially low digestibility forages such as tropical pastures (both green and mature), straws and other crop residues and agricultural by-products which are generally low in protein.

## Management of Resources to Enhance Forage Productivity

To make dairying economically attractive, milk production and productivity has to be enhanced. This is possible only by making available good quality feed and fodder in adequate quantity. Fodder crops are the cheapest source of feed for livestock. Recently, through research efforts, a few feeding technologies have been developed with higher feed conversion efficiencies and having a potential for commercial manufacture, which can partially help in overcoming feed shortage in tropics and enhance animal productivity.

## Promoting Intensive Fodder Production

In India, the area under fodder cultivation has remained static for the last three decades at 4.1 per cent of the total cultivable land, due to pressure of human population. The only way to increase fodder production is through intensive fodder production, especially using high yielding varieties of fodder crops. Integration of forage legumes improves soil fertility and soil structure and controls soil erosion and thus, helps in the sustainable development of agriculture (Reddy *et al.,* 2008).

## Top Feeds/Tree Leaves can act as Fodder Banks

Species of Leucaena, Glyceridia and Sespenia are excellent multipurpose rather wonder trees and bushes which can regularly provide high quality browse as well as serve as fodder bank. Their cultivation also improves soil fertility and the larger branches provide firewood. These trees can also be planted alongside roads and around ponds and edges of paddy fields, as well as in spaces not suitable for cultivation. Apart from these, many tropical trees like prosopis juliflora and Acacia nilotica could be raised on saline soils with gypsum and farmyard manure and serve as green forage (top feed) for the livestock.

## Encouraging Silvipastoral System and Grassland Development

Although the land base for livestock has been shrinking in Indian, which can be attributed to various kinds of pressures, the possibility still exists to obtain more herbage from about 60 m ha of the country's land area, through silvi-pasture system and better grassland management. An integrated system of agro-forestry system in which legumes, pulses (pigeon pea) and grasses can be show in association with fodder tree like Leucaena leucocephala, can provide fodder without any reduction in pulses yield. Similarly, Guinea grass could successfully be grown under coconut plantation, or pasture grass like stylo or citrus or cowpea can be cultivated in the first few years of plantation of citrus or zizyphus (Reddy *et al.,* 2008).

## Exploiting the Genetic Variability in Nutritional Quality of Straws

A large variation in straw quality exists among cultivars with respect to in vitro and in situ DM digestibility (Capper, 1988). This variation could be as high as 10-15 units, which has been studied in most of the cereal crop residues *viz.* rice, wheat, barley, sorghum and millets. In the crop-livestock sustainable production system, better quality of straw can result in 10 per cent increase in productivity of ruminants. Cereal breeders have often overlooked this point. It is high time that the cereal breeders plan their breeding programs in collaboration with animal nutritionists, and thus, help in improving the economic lot of resource poor farmers.

## Nutritional Evaluation of Forage Resources and Development of Feeding Strategies

Poor quality crop residues are still major source of livestock feed, leaving animals undernourished, which increase their susceptibility to diseases, lowering reproduction efficiency ultimately affecting milk, and meat production for human beings, which is a matter of great concern for the country. It is concerned to develop forage based feeding systems for optimum and efficient productive and reproductive performances in different categories of livestock, development of technology for efficient conservation of surplus green grass/biomass available during rainy season, rumen manipulation and improvement of low grade forages/ roughages for improved livestock production and nutrient (protein and energy) management and monitoring blood minerals status in milch animals fed low grade forages.

## Improving Nutritive Value of Crop Residue by Urea Treatment

Crop residues (wheat straw, rice straw, stovers, *etc.*) characterized by high indigestible fibre due to increased lignification of cellulose. Fermentable energy and protein deficiencies in crop residues coupled with their low digestibility impair intake, ruminal functions, and thus animal productivity. Urea, when used for treatment of straw enhances the nutritional quality of straw in terms of increased nitrogen content, improved palatability and digestibility of straw (Sharma *et al.,* 2004).

## Use of Urea Molasses Mineral Block Licks (UMMB)

Urea molasses mineral block is prepared by mixing urea, molasses, mineral mixture and other ingredients in a suitable proportion. It is a readily available source of energy, protein and minerals for the dairy animal. Supplementing an animal with UMMB would provide adequate quantity of these nutrients and slow ingestion of urea leads to efficient microbial protein production and improved digestibility.

## Use of Densified Complete Feed Block

Concept of densified complete feeds with fibrous crop residues is a noble way to increase the intake and improves the nutrients utilization. A complete feed block has been defined as a system of feeding all ingredients including roughages, processed and mixed uniformly, to be made available *ad lib* to the animals. The feeding of complete feed stabilizes rumen fermentation, minimizes fermentation loss and ensures better ammonia utilization (Prasad *et al.,* 2001). This pattern of rumen fermentation enhances utilization of poor quality roughage and improves the palatability of unconventional feeds.

## Feeding of Bypass Nutrients (Protein and fat)

Dairy animals have four compartments in its stomach. The first and the foremost is rumen' where most of the feed items are degraded. Around 60 to 70 per cent of dietary protein meals fed to animals are degraded to ammonia in the rumen. The bypass fat supplies concentrated form of energy and thus, compensates for the inadequate supply of energy from the original diet. The sufficient energy supply boosts up milk production in energy limiting animals. The increase in milk yield is from 10- 25 per cent (Thakur and Shelke, 2010).

## Encouraging the Use of Area Specific Mineral Mixture

Minerals are required by dairy animals for their metabolic functions, growth, milk production, reproduction and health. Animal cannot synthesize minerals inside its body and majority of the feeds generally available in India and other tropical countries are deficient in mineral content, especially trace minerals. Surveys conducted recently in different regions of India have clearly brought out two things to the fore. Firstly, that the mineral deficiencies very form region to region and secondly, that the dairy farmers in Indian, by and large, are not aware of the importance of feeding mineral mixture to their animals (Gowda *et al.,* 2008).

## Recommending Selective Use of Feed Additives

Several feed additives (supplements) have been developed for livestock, and some of these are now commercially available in the market. These supplements appear to be promising, but more research trials are required to be conducted at the research centers to see their suitability as well as economic feasibility under field conditions. Probiotic live yeast cultures are especially effective in enhancing fibre digestion in a situation, where high concentrate feeding is pursued. The technology is more likely to be useful for animals getting low-fibre high-concentrate diets, whereas in the tropical countries, the majority of resource poor farmers are using straw based diets for feeding of bovine stock.

## Reducing Methane Emission through Dietary Interventions

The conditions under which the high density ruminant stock is reared in India and other tropical countries, are conducive for release of high levels of methane from enteric/rumen fermentation into the atmosphere. It calls for making efforts to reduce these levels of emission through technical intervention such as supplementation, fibre fortications and fibre polarization (Padmakumar, 2008). Lately, some herbal extracts, including the supplements containing spices like fenugreek seeds and garlic extracts have been shown to have some positive effect on rumen metabolism, including the defaunation and ruminal methane reduction (Bhatta *et al.,* 2013).

## Conclusion

In the tropical countries, feed shortage, especially the shortage of quality feeds is a serious problem. For increasing the supply of green herbage, the strategies needed are: conservation of degraded pasturelands and development of wastelands, even introducing shrubs and trees, to provide top feeds for livestock. Feeding strategies for ruminants in tropics should also include environmental protection, through reduced methane emission, apart from increasing the productivity of ruminant stock. Some feeding technologies are commercially available today, *viz.* feeding of bypass nutrients and densified TMR, which can boost up the productivity of ruminant stock and also reduce methane emission.

## REFERENCES

Bhatta, R., Saravanan, M., Baruah, L., Sampath, K.T., and Prasad C.S. (2013). Effect of plant secondary compounds on *in vitro* methane, ammonia production and ruminal protozoa population. *J Appl Microbiol.,* **115**(2): 455-65.

Capper, B.S. (1988). Genetic variation in the feeding value of cereal straw. *Anim. Feed Sci. Technol.* **21**,127-140.

Gowda, N.K.S., Prasad, C.S., Selvaraju, S., Reddy, I.J., Ananthram, K. and Sampath,

K.T. (2008). Feeding practices and nutrient status of dairy cows in adopted villages under institute village linkage programme. *Indian Vet. J.,* **85**: 745- 748.

Padmakumar,V. (2008). Livestock, livelihood and environment: The policy context and challenges. *XXXVI Dairy Industry Conference,* BHU,pp. 50-56.

Prasad, C. S., Gowda, N. K. S. and Rammana, J.V. (2001). Feeding strategies to enhance animal productivity. *In; Proceedings of the Xth Animal Nutrition Conference, NDRI, Karnal, India,* pp. 23-45.

Reddy, D. V., Elanchezhian, (2008). Evaluation of tropical tree leaves as ruminant feedstuff based on cell contents, cell wall fractions and polyphenolic compounds. *Livest. Res. Rural Dev.,* **20** (5): 77.

Sharma, K., Dutta, N. and Naulia, U. (2004). An on-farm appraisal of feeding urea-treated straw to buffaloes during late pregnancy and lactation in a mixed farming system. *Livest. Res. Rural Dev.* **16**(11).

Thakur, S.S. and Shelke, S.K. (2010). Effect of supplementing bypass fat prepared from soybean acid oil on milk yield and nutrient utilization in Murrah buffaloes. *Indian J. Anim. Sci.,* **80** (4): 354-357.

## Chapter 3

# Strategic Supplementation of Minerals on Building Economics of Dairy Production in Rural Areas

*Ankur Khare, R.P.S. Baghel, Sunil Nayak, Pramod Sharma and Nagendra Uikey*

*Department of Animal Nutrition,*
*College of Veterinary Science and Animal Husbandry,*
*Nanaji Deshmukh Veterinary Science University, Jabalpur, Madhya Pradesh*

Livestock production is backbone of Indian economy and source of employment in rural areas for centuries. Ruminants play a major role in providing nutritional and livelihood security for millions of rural households in India. Livestock farming is crucially important for provision of animal-based food products for the population and as a source of income for many resource poor farmers in developing countries. With the increase in human population and economic growth of many countries, the demand for livestock products is likely to double in the coming twenty years. However, the main constraint to livestock development in these countries is the scarcity and fluctuation in the quality and quantity of the animal feed supply (Makkar, 2006).

As per 19$^{th}$ livestock census (2012), India has 512 million livestock population. Top 5 states in India having highest livestock population are Uttar Pradesh (68.7 M), Rajasthan (57.7 M), Andhra Pradesh (56.0 M), Madhya Pradesh (36.3 M) and Maharashtra (32.4 M). The ratio of rural to urban livestock population in India is 24.1:1 (19$^{th}$ livestock census, 2012).

## The Availability of Minerals to Animals

The evaluation of feeds and feed supplements as sources of minerals depends not only on the total mineral content or concentration but also on how much can be absorbed from the gut and used by the animals' cells and tissues. This in turn, depends on:

i) The age and species of the animals.

ii) The intake of the mineral relative to the need.

iii) The chemical form in which the mineral is ingested.

iv) The amounts and proportions of other dietary components with which it interacts metabolically.

v) Environmental factors like the accessibility and intensity of sunlight (Ammerman *et al.,* 1995).

## Minerals: The Need for Strategic Supplementation

Mineral supplementation is needed to correct deficiencies in animal diets. Supplementation of minerals is considered to be the least cost way for augmenting productivity especially in grazing ruminants. Organized farming systems make use of compound feeds which contain mineral supplements and hence, do seldom suffer from mineral inadequacy. Samples of compound feeds collected from different states and analyzed in various laboratories in India would support this statement (Table 3.2). This is also the reason for not experiencing mineral deficiency disorders in most of the poultry and swine operations. Nevertheless, the discussion in the previous sections indicate that the grazing ruminants are most prone to deficiency of one or more mineral elements since the forage they graze on hardly supply an adequate amount of minerals the animals require for different productive and

**Table 3.1. Concentration of some Major (per cent) and Trace Elements (ppm) in Compound Livestock Feed in India**

| *State* | *Ca* | *P* | *Ca:P* | *Mg* | *Cu* | *Zn* | *Fe* | *Mn* |
|---|---|---|---|---|---|---|---|---|
| Critical level | <0.3 | <0.25 | 2:1 | <02 | <8.0 | <30.0 | <50.0 | <40.0 |
| Assam[1] | 0.76 | - | - | 0.47 | 5.6 | 22.6 | 93 | 38.6 |
| Gujarat[2] | 0.66 | 134 | - | 0.67 | 20.5 | 192 | 1032 | 146.1 |
| Himachal Pradesh | 0.93 | 1.00 | 0.93 | - | 13.9 | 51.6 | - | - |
| Karnataka[3] | 0.98 | 1.51 | 0.65 | 0.68 | 12.6 | 39.4 | 508 | - |
| Kerala[4] | 0.98 | 0.92 | 1.06 | 0.58 | 16.3 | 49.3 | 828 | - |
| Rajasthan[5] | 0.76 | 1.11 | 0.68 | 0.64 | 25.9 | 106.1 | 829 | 105.9 |
| West Bengal[6] | 1.4 | 0.9 | 1.7 | - | 5.4 | 25.9 | 431 | 87.1 |

*Source: 1: Buragohain et al., 2006; 2: Garg et al., 2003; 3: Gowda et al., 2002; 4: ICAR Net Work Project on Micronutrients in Animal Nutrition and Production, Trissur Center, Kerala (1999); 5: Garg et al., 2005; 6: ICAR Net Work Project on Micronutrients in Animal Nutrition and Production, Kolkata Center, West Bengal (2004).*

reproductive purposes. The situation gets confounded and rather aggravated because of the supplementation strategy adopted by the animal owners and interestingly the situation is almost similar across the country.

**Table 3.2. Major (per cent) and Trace (ppm) Element Concentration in Dry and Green Roughages in India**

| | *Ca* | *P* | *Ca:P* | *Mg* | *Cu* | *Zn* | *Fe* | *Mn* |
|---|---|---|---|---|---|---|---|---|
| **Critical level** | **<0.3** | **025** | **2:1** | **<02** | **8.0** | **<30** | **<50** | **<40** |
| **Mineral content of straw (include paddy, maize and bajra straw)** | | | | | | | | |
| Assam | 0.63 | - | - | 0.44 | 7.2 | 21.4 | 122.3 | 43.6 |
| Kerala | 026 | 0.09 | 2.9 | 021 | 10.0 | 55.0 | 866.4 | - |
| Himachal Pradesh | 0.09 | 0.03 | 3.0 | - | 1.9 | 15.8 | - | - |
| Rajasthan | 028 | 0.09 | 3.1 | 0.21 | 6.0 | 28.6 | 356.4 | 168.2 |
| Haryana | 031 | 0.12 | 2.6 | - | 26.0 | 14.5 | 176.0 | 16.5 |
| West Bengal | | | | | | | | |
| Coastal soil | 0.12 | 0.06 | 2.0 | - | 7.4 | 29.0 | 226.4 | 272.8 |
| Laterite soil | 0.15 | 0.04 | 3.8 | - | 10.6 | 32.3 | 262.5 | 22.3 |
| Alluvial soil | 0.13 | 0.06 | 2.2 | - | 8.3 | 41.1 | 224.4 | 23.9 |
| Calculated mean | 0.25 | 0.06 | 2.43 | 028 | 9.7 | 29.7 | 319.2 | 91.2 |
| **Mineral content of green roughage (include pasture grass and non leguminous cultivated fodder)** | | | | | | | | |
| Assam | 0.6 | - | - | 0.06 | 24.3 | 24.3 | 330.8 | 109.9 |
| Kerala | 0.3 | 0.2 | 1.4 | 022 | 10.2 | 48.6 | 627.2 | . |
| Himachal Pradesh | 0.53 | 0.19 | 2.8 | 0.19 | 10.8 | 30.4 | 365 | 60.8 |
| Rajasthan | 0.87 | 022 | 4.0 | 0.62 | 11.5 | 30.4 | 422 | 92.3 |
| Haryana | 1.56 | 0.19 | 8.2 | - | 28.5 | 24.1 | 342 | 38.0 |
| West Bengal | | | | | | | | |
| Coastal soil | 0.42 | 0.17 | 2.5 | - | 53.01 | 42.63 | 403.53 | 35.66 |
| Laterite soil | 0.49 | 021 | 2.3 | - | 62 | 22.7 | 323.1 | 71.8 |
| Alluvial soil | 0.42 | 026 | 1.6 | - | 4.9 | 24.9 | 297.8 | 78.9 |
| Calculated mean | 0.65 | 0.18 | 2.85 | 027 | 18.7 | 31.0 | 388.9 | 69.6 |

The data presented in Table 3.3 is a clear revelation of macro and micro mineral status of the dry and green roughages in Indian condition. The data are almost a national representation and are collected across the country from different agro climatic and soil conditions. Interestingly, the data is not too widely dispersed and the coefficient of variation (not shown) is found to be insignificant.

The table brings into fore the following facts:

- ☆ There exists almost moderate to severe deficiency of Ca and P in dry roughage.

- Moderate deficiency with regards to P is there in green roughage.
- Trace elements are adequate in dry and green roughage though Cu is just marginal in the dry roughages in most of the samples in the surveyed areas.
- Fe concentration is much above the minimum critical level and its supplementation seems to be unnecessary.

**Table 3.3. A Good Tree Choice Mineral Supplements**

| | |
|---|---|
| 1. | Contains a minimum of 6-8 per cent total P. In areas where forages are consistently lower than 0.2 *per cent* P, mineral supplements in the 8-10 per cent P range are preferred. |
| 2. | Has a Ca:P ratio not substantially over 2:1 |
| 3. | Provides a significant proportion (*i.e.* about 50 per cent) of the trace element requirements for Co, Cu, I, Mn, Zn and Se if required. Fe is not needed in most circumstances. |
| 4. | Is sufficiently palatable to allow close to adequate consumption in relation to requirements. |
| 5. | Has an acceptable particle size that will allow adequate mixing without smaller size particles settling out. |
| 6. | Is formulated for the area involved, the level of animal productivity, and the environment in which it will be fed and is as economical as possible. |

To assess how the mineral status of feeds and fodder affect the mineral balance in grazing ruminants Das *et al.* (2003) conducted a survey in two different agro-climatic regions of West Bengal.

## Need for the Area Specific Mineral Supplementation

It has already been emphasized repeatedly that it is the ruminants that depend predominantly on forages do require mineral supplementation as they seldom receive adequate supplies of particular minerals because of moderate to sever deficiencies of one or more mineral elements in dry and green roughages. The problem is not so drastic in the organized farm sector or in the poultry and swine operations (McDowell, 1985) and hence, our discussion will focus on the need of the grazing ruminants (Table 3.4).

Prior to opt for the supplementation a few points need to be assessed and assured.

- The distribution of the mineral elements in the soil and local feed resources.
- The existence of the practice of mineral supplementation in the area concerned.
- The average productivity of animals in the said area.
- Calculation of the mineral requirement of the animals.

- ☆ Formulation of the mineral mixture containing all the elements needed by the animals.
- ☆ Finally, fortification of the diet with the said mineral mixture.

Free Choice mineral supplement: Free-choice mineral supplements are generally considered only for livestock that do not have access to concentrates, as minerals for those receiving concentrates are generally provided as part of the concentrate mixture. As a low-cost insurance complete mineral supplements should be available to grazing livestock free choice (McDowell 1985). A "good" free choice mineral supplement should have the following characteristic features:

**Table 3.4. Relative Bioavailability of some Major and Trace Elements**

| *Element* | *Source* | *Reference Compound* | *Relative Bioavailability Per cent* |
|---|---|---|---|
| Calcium | Ca carbonate | . | 40-57 |
| | Bone meal | Ca carbonate | 63-138 |
| | Ca chloride | Ca carbonate | 71-132 |
| | Calcite | Ca carbonate | 49 |
| | Di calcium phosphate | Ca carbonate | 56-126 |
| Phosphorus | Bone meal | Di calcium phosphate | 30 |
| | Di calcium phosphate | | 33-85 |
| | Rock phosphate | Di calcium phosphate | 17-54 |
| | Defluorinated phosphate | Di calcium phosphate | 29-85 |
| Zinc | Zinc sulfate | Zinc oxide | 100 |
| | Zinc chloride | Zinc oxide | 42 |
| | Zinc carbonate | Zinc oxide | 58 |
| | Zinc methionine | Zinc oxide | 103-133 |
| Manganese | Manganese carbonate | Mn sulfate | 2046 |
| | Manganese oxide | Mn sulfate | 25-39 |
| | Manganese methionine | Mn sulfate | 102-157 |

*Source*: Ammerman *et al.* (1995).

## Organic Minerals

A new age supplementation strategy: The key to the effectiveness of a mineral supplement is not necessarily its biological availability, but its biological activity. Traditionally, inorganic salts such as oxides, sulfates and carbonates have been added to the diet to provide the desired amount to meet the requirements of the animals. These are broken down to varying extents during digestion to 'free' ions' and are then absorbed. However, they may also complex to other dietary molecules and become difficult to absorb or, if completely complexed, totally unavailable to the animal. Thus, the availability of the element may vary substantially.

## Economic Aspects of Chelated and Proteinate Forms of Trace Elements

Economic response is the key concern. Chelated minerals cost 10 to 15 times more per milligram of mineral compared to inorganic sources. Commercial chelated mineral programs cost range from 4 cents to 18 cents per cow per day (depending on the combination and level of chelated minerals selected). Two approaches are listed below:

1. Supplement one-third of selected trace minerals as chelated mineral (400 g of zinc as organic zinc) and two-thirds as inorganic mineral (800 g of zinc as zinc sulfate for example).
2. Feed recommended levels (Table 3.5) as inorganic minerals (1200 g as zinc as zinc sulfate) plus an additional 25 per cent as chelated zinc (300 g of zinc as organic zinc for example).

**Table 3.5. Economics of Milk Production in the Dairy after Supplementation**

| *Treat-ment* | *Roughage Fed (kg)* | *Cost of Roughage (Rs)* | *Conc. Fed (kg)* | *Cost of Conc (Rs)* | *Total Feeding Cost (Rs)* | *Misc. Exp. (Rs)* | *Total Cost (Rs)* | *Milk Yield (lit)* | *Cost of Feed/ kg Milk (Rs)* |
|---|---|---|---|---|---|---|---|---|---|
| I | 19.34 | 13.05 | 9.00 | 75.75 | 88.80 | 3 | 91.80 | 7.48 | 12.27 |
| II | 18.42 | 12.43 | 9.00 | 75.75 | 88.18 | 3 | 91.18 | 7.54 | 12.09 |
| III | 19.82 | 13.37 | 7.72 | 64.97 | 78.34 | 3 | 81.34 | 7.23 | 11.25 |
| IV | 19.53 | 13.17 | 7.35 | 61.86 | 75.03 | 3 | 78.03 | 7.18 | 10.86 |

It has been observed that instead of total replacement of inorganic minerals with organically complexed mineral elements, it will always be a more prudent approach to opt for a partial replacement of the conventional inorganic forms of supplemental minerals with the respective organic forms. This will save the economy of the farmers and will promote the productivity at the same time.

## Supplementation Strategy

While formulating die supplementation strategy some factors need to be remembered:

***Plant maturity:*** As plants mature, mineral contents decline and hence the need for mineral supplementation increases when a dry or drought condition prevails for a while in a year.

***Energy-protein supplements:*** Protein and energy supplements that also provide minerals decrease both the need and desire for free choice minerals.

***Individual requirements:*** The level of productivity and the physiological condition like gestation and lactation of an animal influence the mineral need.

## Supplementation Strategy for Grazing Ruminants Receiving No Concentrate

Animals that primarily depend on pasture have different supplementation needs than those receiving concentrates. Free choice mineral mixture or a mineral lick is the preferred option to supplement these animals. A urea-molasses-mineral block would be an effective strategy to supplement a protein substitute and the mineral simultaneously especially when the quality of the forage is poor. P is generally limiting and hence a free choice mineral mixture containing adequate Ca, P, common salt and selected trace elements is needed to be supplied. Fe is always an excess in most of the agro-climatic zones of India and need not to be supplemented. Areas having deficient Se require its supplementation while those (like the northern plains encompassing Punjab, Haryana, upper Uttar Pradesh and Rajasthan) showing toxic levels of Se need sulfur in the mineral premix as the antagonist of Se.

## Supplementation Strategy for Grazing Ruminants Receiving Concentrate

The best means of providing minerals to ruminants receiving concentrates would be to combine the minerals with the concentrate diet, including Ca, P, and a trace mineralized salt (NaCl plus Co, Cu, I, Mn, Se and Zn depending on local need). Fe may be included if condition deserves for. The less dietary forage intake, the higher level of Ca and P is required. S may be added to the premix if non-protein nitrogen is added to the concentrate. The balance of individual minerals is important in this regard to ensure proper absorption and utilization of the minerals.

In organized farming sector as well, the most common method to deliver trace minerals to dairy cattle has been trace mineralized salt. Feed tags must be carefully reviewed to determine the level (mg per day) that is being offered and if the mineral form is biologically available. Customized trace mineral premixtures are becoming more common because they can be formulated to balance mineral profiles and meet mineral needs depending on the farm condition. Forage testing is recommended for Zn, Cu and Mn and if conditions desire then Fe as well on an annual basis to establish herd micromineral profiles, evaluate feed changes, and avoid/correct mineral imbalances.

Baghel *et al.* (2011) conducted a study in rural areas of Jabalpur district of Madhya Pradesh to study the feeding regime of lactating anoestrous buffaloes. Data was collected through the survey of the Bhamnoda village near Jabalpur. Study revealed that most of the animals in the village were deficient in nutrients (protein and energy), macro minerals (calcium and phosphorus) and trace minerals (cobalt, copper, zinc, manganese and iron). Strategic supplement was prepared using deficient nutrients and was supplemented to the buffaloes. The results revealed that there was increase in milk production within the range of 5.0-14.0 per cent. The net profit per day per animal to farmers ranged between

Rs. 1.50-10.14. Supplementation of trace minerals also improved the onset of estrous and conception rate in animals.

## REFERENCES


Adams, S.N. and Honeysett J.L. (1964) *Austr. J. Agricu. Res.,* **15:** 357-367.

Ammerman, C.B., Baker, D.H. and Lewis, A.J. (1995). Bioavailability of nutrients for animals. *Academic Press, New York.*

Arthur, J.R. (1992). *Proc. Nutr. Soc. Australia,* **17**: 91-98.

Buragohain, R., Ghosh, M.K., Baruah, K.K., Pathak, P.K. and Bhattacharya, M. (2006). *Anim. Nutr. Feed Technol.,* **6**: 289-294.

Coates, D.B., Kerridge, P.C., Miller, C.P. and Winter, W.H. (1990). *Trop. Grassland,* **24**: 209-220.

Das, A., Ghosh, T.K. and Haidar, S. (2003). *Indian J. Anim. Sci.,* **73**: 448-454.

Fordyce, F.M., Masara, D. and Appleton, J.D. (1996). Stream sediment, soil and forage chemistry as predictors of cattle mineral status in north east Zimbabwe. In: *Environmental Geochemistry and Health.* (Appleton J.D., Fuge R. and McCall GH.J., eds.) *Geological Society Special Publication No.* **113**, London, pp. 23-37.

Garg, M.R., Bhanderi, B.M. and Sherasia, P.L. (2003). *Anim. Nutr. Feed Technol.,* **3**: 179-188.

Garg, M.R., Bhanderi, B.M. and Sherasia, P.L. (2005). *Anim. Nutr. Feed Technol.,* **5**: 9- 20.

Gowda, N.K.S., Prasad, C.S., Ramana, J.V. and Shivaramaiah, M.T. (2002). *Indian J. Anim. Sci.,* **72**: 165-170.

Hopkins, A. Adamson, A.H. and Bowling, P.J. (1994). *Grass Forage Sci.,* **49**: 9-20 Jones R.J. (1990). *Trop. Grasslands,* **24**: 131-139.

Kundu, B. (2004). Studies on trace element supplementation on nutritional and reproductive performance of dairy cattle in the red and laterite agro-climatic zones of West Bengal. Ph.D. Thesis submitted to the West Bengal University of Animal and Fishery Sciences, Kolkata, India.

McDowell, L.R. (1985). Minerals in animal and human nutrition (Tony J Cunha ed.). *Academic Press, New York.*

Minson, D.J. (1990). Forages in ruminant nutrition. Academic Press, San Diego, California, pp. 208-229.

Morillo D., McDowell L.R., Chicco C.F., Perdomo J.T., Conrad J.H. and Martin F.G (1989) *Nutr. Reports International,* 39: 1247-1262.

Pastrana, R., McDowell, L.R., Conrad, J.H. and Wilkinson, N.S. (1991). *Small Rumin. Res.,* **5**: 9-21.

Philippo M. (1983). The role of dose response trials in predicting trace element disorders. In: *Trace Elements in Animal Production in* Veterinary *Practice.* (Suttle N.F., Gunn R.G, Allen W.M., Linklater K.A. and Wiener G eds.). British Society of Animal Production Special Publication No. 7, Edinburgh, pp. 51- 60.

Prabowo, A., McDowell L.R., Wilkinson N.S., Wilcox C.J. and Conrad J.A. (1990). *Buffalo J.,* **1**: 17-32.

Underwood, E.J. and Suttle, N.F. (1999). The Mineral Nutrition of Livestock (3rd edition). *CABI Publishing, London.*

Valdes, J.L., McDowell, L.R. and Koger, M. (1988). *J. Prod. Agric.,* **1**: 351-355. Winks, L. (1990). *Trop. Grasslands,* **24**: 140-158.

Chapter 4

# Organic Livestock Production: Challenge for Livestock Feeding

*G.P. Lakhani*

*Department of Livestock Production and Management,*
*College of Veterinary Science and Animal Husbandry,*
*Nanaji Deshmukh Veterinary Science University, Jabalpur, Madhya Pradesh*

## Introduction

There was phenomenal growth in country's milk production during the recent decades has resulted in India emerging as world's largest producer with the annual milk production reaching to the level of 133 million tons in 2012-13 (BAHS 2012-13). However, there has been an increased concern voiced over quality of milk and milk products including the contents of contamination and pollutant and the residual effect of various pesticides, insecticide, chemicals, drugs and hormones. Due to this, the interest in organic dairying is increasing at rapid pace worldwide with faster growth in demand of organic milk and milk products. The word organic' signifies food or farming method practiced without using artificial chemicals *i.e.* something natural and inherently good. Sir Albert Howard is widely considered to be the "father of organic farming".The Government of India has launched the National Programme for Organic Production (NPOP) in the year 2001.

## What is Organic Farming?

The term *conventional farming'* refers to a production system which employs a full range of pre- and post-plant tillage practices (*e.g.* plough, disc plant, and cultivator), synthetic fertilizers, pesticides and insecticides. It is characterized by a high degree of crop specialization.

The term *Organic farming* is a production system which avoids the use of synthetic fertilizers, pesticides; insecticides, growth regulators, and livestock feed additives. The basic objectives of organic farming are environmental, social, and economic sustainability.

According to the International Federation of Organic Agriculture Movement (Willer *et al.,* 2008), the major objectives of organic farming include:

1. Production of high quality food in sufficient quantity in harmony with natural systems and cycles.
2. Enhancing biological cycles within the farming system involving micro-organisms, soil flora and fauna, plants and animals.
3. Maintaining long-term soil fertility and genetic diversity of the production system and its surroundings including plant and wildlife.
4. Promoting healthy use with proper care of water resources and all life there in.
5. Creating harmonious balance between crop production and animal husbandry.
6. Minimizing all forms of pollution.

Livestock can make an important contribution to an organic farming system by improving and maintaining the fertility of the soil, maintaining the flora through grazing, enhancing biodiversity and facilitating complementary interactions in the farm.

## Characteristics of Organic Livestock Production Systems

Organic livestock management shall aim to utilize natural breeding methods, minimize stress, prevent disease, progressively eliminate the use of chemical allopathic veterinary drugs (including antibiotics), and maintain animal health and welfare. Better management practices and prevention of illness are emphasized over treatment. Animals are marketed as having been raised without the use of persistent toxic pesticides, antibiotics or parasiticides (Von Borrel and Sorensen, 2004).

Thus, the primary characteristics of organic livestock production systems are:

1. No routine use of growth promoters, animal offal, prophylactic antibiotics or any other additives.
2. Organic livestock should be fed on organically produced grass, fodder and other feed, without the use of artificial fertilizers or pesticides on crops or grass.
3. Animals living conditions which will allow them to perform the basic aspects of their innate behavior.

4. Animals should not be kept in confined spaces where they cannot carry out their natural behavior such as standing and moving around. Housing should satisfy the needs of the animals concerned. Livestock must have access to free range exercise area and/or grazing apart from specified exemptions.
5. Adequate ventilation, light, space and comfort to permit ample freedom of movement to develop the animal's natural social behavior.
6. Breeds should be chosen to suit local needs and local conditions and resources.
7. There should not be consumption of genetically modified organism and products.
8. Animal health management should be mainly based on prevention. There is preventive use of chemically synthesized medication (allopathic medicines). Emphasis must be given on use of herbal, naturopathic and homeopathic treatments.
9. Sick and injured animals must be treated immediately as well being of the animal is more important (although this may affect their status with regards to organic certification).

## Advantages of Organic Dairy Farming

1. Well-managed organic dairy farms are less harmful to the environment than conventional dairies, and there is evidence that the milk they produce may be better for our health.
2. Consumers are catching on to these advantages: demand for organic dairy products has risen quickly in recent years.
3. Milk contains Conjugated Linoleic Acid (CLA). Function of CLA in human body is to boost immune system and reduce the growth of tumors.CLA levels in organic milk are higher because these cows eat greater amounts of grass, hay and silage (McBride and Greene, 2009).
4. Avoid environmental pollution.
5. Show lower presence of pesticide residue in organic milk, although organic milk may not be completely pesticide free. A possible presence of pesticide residue in food may be due to environmental contaminants.
6. Organic milk is free from the presence of antibiotic residues which reduces the chance of development of microbial resistance.
7. Organic milk is produced without the use of synthetic hormones, so their residue is not present in milk.
8. Animals managed in conventional system in confinement contribute to manure with a high methane producing capacity. In contrast cattle raised in pasture, eating a more natural, low-energy diet composed of grasses

and other forages, produce manure with about half of the potential to generate methane.

## Challenges to Organic Farming

Despite serious efforts of some NGO's, it appears that India is lagging far behind in the adoption of organic farming. For laying the spadework for the spread of organic agriculture in the country, certain issues require attention at the government policymaking levels. These include:

1. Substantial financial support by the governments to promote organic farming;
2. Market development for the sale of organic products;
3. Simplification of the process of certification;
4. Reduction in certification cost.
5. A vigorous campaign to highlight the benefits of organic farming against the conventional system to increase awareness of both farmers and consumers

## Objectives of Organic Farming

The major objectives of organic farming include:

1. Production of high quality food in sufficient quantity in harmony with natural systems and cycles.
2. Enhancing biological cycles within the farming system involving micro-organisms, soil flora and fauna, plants and animals.
3. Maintaining long-term soil fertility and genetic diversity of the production system and its surroundings including plant and wildlife.
4. Promoting healthy use with proper care of water resources and all life there in.
5. Creating harmonious balance between crop production and animal husbandry.
6. Minimizing all forms of pollution.

## Concept of Organic Dairy Farming

Organic production systems are based on specific standards precisely formulated for food production and aim at achieving agro ecosystems, which are socially and ecologically sustainable. It is based on minimizing the use of external inputs through use of on-farm resources efficiently compared to industrial agriculture.

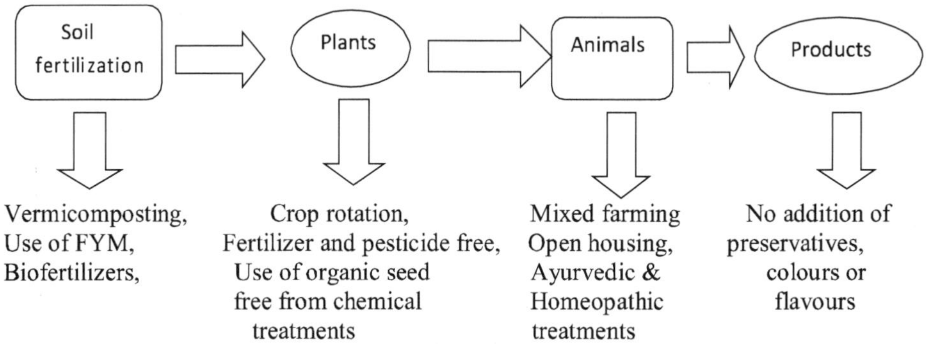


## Importance of Organic Dairy Farming

Today, the burgeoning population pressure has forced many countries to use chemicals and fertilizers to increase the farm productivity for meeting their ever-increasing food requirements. Thus, prolong usage of chemicals has, however, resulted in human and soil health hazards along with environmental pollution. Farmers in the developed countries are therefore, being encouraged to convert their existing farms into organic farm.

Consumption of genetically modified (GM) products, fears of pesticides, insecticides, fertilizers, chemicals, antibiotics, and other medicinal residue in non-organic food and generalized belief that the organic products are more nutritious, healthy and tasty and potential scope of high-value niche market for small scale farmer and entrepreneurs (Kamboj and Parsad, 2013).

## Scope of Organic Livestock Farming in India

Under Indian condition, Organic Livestock Farming is most suitable because of Indigenous technical knowledge and practices followed by Indian farmers. India has a strong traditional farming system with innovative farmers, vast dry lands and least use of chemicals. In fact, the rain fed tribal, north-east and hilly regions of the country where negligible chemicals are used in agriculture have been practicing subsistence agriculture for a long period; such areas are organic by default (Butterworth *et al.*, 2003; Reddy, 2010b). In India only 30 per cent of total cultivable area is covered with fertilizers where irrigation facilities are available and in the remaining 70 per cent of arable land, which is mainly rain-fed, negligible amount of fertilizers is being used. Farmers in these areas often use organic manure as a source of nutrients that are readily available either in their own farm or in their locality. India has around 1,426 certified organic farms, which produces approximately 14,000 tons of output annually (Chadrashekar, 2010).

## Why Organic Farming?

In recent years, there is a lot of debate between the proponents of organic farming and a section of the community who questioned the scientific validity and feasibility of organic farming (Chhonkar, 2003). The most often debated issues on organic farming fall under the following six categories:

1. Can organic farming produce enough food for everybody?
2. Is it possible to meet the nutrient requirements of crops entirely from organic sources?
3. Are there any significant environmental benefits of organic farming?
4. Is the food produced by organic farming superior in quality?
5. Is organic agriculture economically feasible?
6. Is it possible to manage pests and diseases in organic farming?.

## How Organic Milk is Superior?

The level of conjugated lenoleic acid (CLA) which is one of the beneficial fatty acid was 60 per cent higher in organic milk than in conventional milk. A Study shows that the cow that ate grass and clover instead of grain exhibited higher levels of CLA, alpha linoleic acid (ALA), alpha tocopherol (vitamin E) and three carotenoids (beta- caroten, lutein and zeaxathin) in their milk than conventionally reared cow (Kamboj and Prasad, 2013).

## Characteristics of an Ideal Organic Livestock Farm

Animal health and well-being through better living conditions, improved welfare measures and good feeding practices are ensured through a set of standards and

the maintenance of written records by organic livestock farmers. Better management practices and prevention of illness are emphasized over treatment.

Thus, the primary characteristics of organic livestock production systems are:

1. Well-defined standards and practices which can be verified.
2. Greater attention to animal welfare.
3. No routine use of growth promoters, animal offal, prophylactic antibiotics or any other additives.
4. At least 80 per cent of the animal feed grown according to organic standards, without the use of artificial fertilizers or pesticides on crops or grass.

To be precise, organic meat, milk and eggs are produced, harvested, preserved and processed according to verified organic standards. Practically speaking, organic methods call for a change in existing production systems.

Organic livestock farming is not a production method meant to solve all problems in livestock production. It is primarily a production method for a specific premium market, demanding high quality standards during the entire production process, advanced management qualifications and certification standard.

## Certification Bodies in India

In India, Agricultural Processed Foods Export Development Authority (APEDA) under Ministry of Commerce is the controlling body for organic certification. Currently 11 certification/accredited agencies have been authorized to undertake certification process in India under National Programme for Organic Production (NPOP).

1. BVQI (India) Pvt. Ltd., Mumbai
2. Ecocert SA, Aurangabad
3. IMO Control Private Limited, Bangalore
4. Indian Organic Certification Agency (INDOCERT), Cochin
5. International Resources for Fairer Trade (IRFT), Mumbai
6. Lacon Quality Certification Pvt. Ltd, Thiruvalla
7. Natural Organic Certification Association (NOCA), Pune
8. One Cert Asia Agri Certification Private Limited, Jaipur
9. SGS India Pvt. Ltd., Gurgaon
10. Skal International, Bangalore
11. Uttaranchal State Organic Certification Agency (USOCA), Dehradun

## Process of Certification

In order to certify a farm, the farmer is typically required to engage in a number of new activities, in addition to normal farming operations, study the organic standards, compliance farm facilities of production method must comply with standards, documentation, planning, inspection, fee and record keeping written day to day farming records.

## Conversion Period

The time between the start of organic management and certification of animal husbandry is known as the conversion period. The whole farm, including livestock, should be converted according to the standards over a period of three years.

## Duration of Conversion Period

Animal products may be sold as "product of organic agriculture" only after the farm or relevant part of it has been under conversion for at least one year and in case of dairy and egg production, this period shall not be less than 30 days. Animals present on the farm at the time of conversion may be sold for organic meat if the organic standards have been followed for one year.

## Salient Features in Organic Dairy Farming

Some key considerations in organic animal husbandry that producers and other stakeholders need to take into account are listed below:

## A. Origin of Livestock

All livestock and livestock products that are sold, labeled or advertised as organic must be raised under continuous organic management from the last third of gestation or at hatching.

## B. Livestock Feed

The total ration of livestock that are produced under organic management must consist of agricultural products that have been organically produced and handled organically. This includes pasture, forage and crops. Avoid use of plastic pellets, urea, manure and by-products from mammalian or poultry slaughter are not allowed.

## C. Living Condition and Regulation for Organic Dairy Farming

An organic livestock producer must create and maintain living conditions that promote the health and accommodate the natural behaviour of the animal. These living conditions must include access to the outdoors, shade, shelter, fresh air, direct sunlight for particular species and access pastures for ruminants. Following living condition considered as:

- ☆ Round the year access for all animals to the outdoors, shade, shelter, exercise areas, fresh air, clean water for drinking, and direct sunlight suitable to the species.
- ☆ During the grazing season suitable pasture for livestock.
- ☆ Appropriate clean, dry bedding free from dust and dirt.
- ☆ Appropriate shelter designed should allow for livestock.
- ☆ Natural maintenance, comfort behaviors, and opportunity to exercise.
- ☆ Suitable environmental conditions.
- ☆ Sufficient feeding space without crowding and without competition for food and Continuous indoor confinement in yards and feeding space are prohibited.

## D. Waste Management

Organic livestock producers are mandated to manage manure so that it does not contribute to the contamination of crops, soil or water and optimizes the recycling of nutrients.

## E. Health Care Regulation for Organic Dairy and Livestock

Organic livestock production requires producers to establish preventive health care practices. These practices include:

1. Selecting the appropriate type and species of livestock.
2. Creating an appropriate environment that minimizes stress, disease condition and parasites infection.

3. Proper vaccination schedule and veterinary biologics.
4. Standard animal husbandry practices to promote animal well-being.

## F. Record Keeping

Organic livestock operations need to maintain records for a number of reasons such as:

1. For the financial management of any organic livestock enterprise.
2. To verify the organic status of the animals and the production, harvesting and handling practices associated with them and their products.
3. These records must demonstrate compliance with the Organic Food Production Act in India and equivalent legislation elsewhere.

So keeping a record is essential because organic production generally requires more record keeping than conventional production (Willer and Kilcher, 2011).

## Breeds and Breeding

Organic farming prefers to the use of local, native and pure breeds.

- ☆ Breeds should be able to adapt to local condition in terms of its disease resistance, maintenance and adaptability.
- ☆ Good milk producer
- ☆ Good mothering ability, hardiness and thriftiness and ability to forage under organic environment.
- ☆ Local desi cattle can be up-graded if necessary.
- ☆ High feed intake should be there when raising heifers.
- ☆ The indigenous cattle and buffaloes in India is ideal for organic system.

## Conclusions

In order to make organic dairy farming success there is need to take care of certain points, like reducing the paper work and cost for certification; sourcing of organic inputs like feeds and fodder, disease prevention, cost of production and maintaining animal health *etc.* These can be insured by organic production methods. Organic farming can provide quality food without adversely affecting the soil's health and the environment. It should not necessarily be interpreted to mean that the foods produced are healthier, safer or all natural. It simply means that the products follow the defined standard of production and handling, although surveys indicate that consumers consider the organic label as an indication of purity and careful handling.

Chapter 5

# Contract Livestock Farming: A Possible Solution for Multilayer Problems in Animal Husbandry

*Biswajit Roy*

*Department of Livestock Production and Management,*
*College of Veterinary Science and Animal Husbandry,*
*Nanaji Deshmukh Veterinary Science University, Jabalpur, Madhya Pradesh*

## Introduction

Agriculture is mainstay of the Indian economy. The share of agriculture and allied sectors in GVA (gross value added) declined from 18.2 per cent in 2012-13 to 16.4 per cent in 2017-18. However, the declining share does not undermine the significance of the sector for employment, livelihood and food security. Further, the agriculture sector itself has been witnessing a gradual structural change in recent years. The share of livestock in GVA of agriculture has been rising since 2011-12, while that of the crop sector declined from 65 per cent in 2011-12 to 60 per cent in 2015-16 (Economic Survey, 2017-18). The livestock sector has important role in Indian economy and also there is a need to improve the present stage of livestock sector further. Livestock production has been steadily growing, faster than any other subsector. There are a number of constraints confronting the livestock production and impedes its growth and development. Some of the important aspects are discussed below:

a) **Shortage of feeds and fodder:** Forage based economical feeding strategies are required to reduce the cost of quality livestock product as the feed alone constitutes 60-70 per cent of the animal production cost. Thus any attempt towards enhancing feed availability and economizing the feed cost would result in increased margin of profits to livestock owners also. There is tremendous pressure of livestock on available total feed and fodder, as land available for fodder production has been decreasing. At present, the country faces a net deficit of 35.6 per cent green fodder, 10.95 per cent dry crop residues and 44 per cent concentrate feed ingredients (IGFRI, 2013).

b) **Marketing problem:** Marketing involves the conveying of livestock product from farmers to consumers. Some of the problems of marketing affecting the livestock sector include poor transportation means, poor packaging and poor quality.

c) **Poor credit availability:** Inspite of existence of thousands of rural credit institution, regional rural banks and rural branches. Disbursement of loans for livestock sector is almost 5 per cent of the total loan disbursement in agriculture. It is extremely hard to access due to procedural complexity, inordinate delay, high interest rate *etc.* (Birthal and Jha, 2005; Birthal *et al.*, 2006).

d) **Storage and processing:** Most of the livestock products are perishable in nature. The lack of storage and processing facilities affect both national food security and household food security. Even when there is a huge production, because of lack of good storage facilities leads to animal products are unfit for human consumption and ultimately shortage of food from animal origin.

e) **Lack of good infrastructure:** In the rural area where most of the farmers operate without good infrastructure in place, is a major problem, as it affects investment, trade, and agricultural production. This problem persists as most of the government favours urban development over rural development. Lack of infrastructure is one of the limiting factor for investment by the private players in the animal husbandry sector.

f) **Prevalence of diseases:** Animals are susceptible to diseases due to lack of health coverage in remote areas.

g) **Increase cost of production:** Average costs of various inputs used in livestock farming are increasing day by day and create further burden to the farmer.

h) **Shortage of labour :** Shortage of trained and dedicated labour is another hurdle in animal production. This is because of the fact that young generation is not much interested in farming and they migrates to the city for their livelihood. The main cause of this migration is the perception by young men that farm labour cannot support them and their families.

i) **Lack of link between research and extension:** The lack of a close working relationship between national agricultural research and extension organizations, and with different categories of farmers and farm organizations, is one of the most difficult institutional problems. Suitable model or process is required to be implemented to resolve major issues related to the constraint in animal husbandry sector. One such model is contract farming.

## What is Contract Farming?

Contract farming involves a pre-agreed price between the company and the farmer. The agreement is defined by the commitment of the farmer to provide an agricultural commodity of a certain type at a time and a price and in the quantity required by a committed buyer, mostly a large company. The Indian animal production system is undergoing rapid transformation and there is growing evidence that contract farming will have an important role in this transformation. Establishing farm-firm linkages is not only about providing assured markets, reducing risk, and ensuring remunerative' prices, but also providing critical services such as credit, insurance, grading and inspection, technology extension, and market information. These institutional services can help elevate the scale at which small holders can operate, raise their productivity and income, and mitigate the risks involved in participating in markets for high value livestock, and fishery products.

Pig and poultry meat can be produced commercially more cheaply than other meats, so markets for these products derived from landless systems are growing rapidly. In India, poultry birds are mostly reared under contract farming system among the other livestock species. Economies of scale in processing and marketing may be derived by vertical integration of smallholder producers with large-scale urban-based processors and input suppliers or by producer co-operatives. Similar issues arise for intensive smallholder milk producers, who have formed dairy processing cooperatives in countries like India.

## Why Contract Farming in India?

- In India the farmers face the problems of traditional technology and management practices, little bargaining power with input suppliers and produce markets, inadequate infrastructure and market information, poor package of produce and inadequate capital to produce grow a quality produce. They are waiting for change for better living standards.
- Contract farming helps small farmers to participate in the production of high value animals.
- Large areas are required by the animal product processing firm for an intensive animal husbandry to follow a uniform method of animal rearing that would reduce their production and transaction costs with the growers.

- Contract farming will maximise the profits to the farmers and minimise risk in farming like production related risks, transfer price risk and produce risk.
- The farmers find it easy to get under one roof inputs, technological and extension services and more importantly, the marketing of their produce with assured cash returns.
- Contract farming facilitates more and more private Companies to develop backward linkages with the farmers.
- Access to animal husbandry loans at attractive terms through tie-ups with Banks is facilitated through contract farming.

## Advantages of Contract Farming

### For Farmers

- Inputs and production services are often supplied by the sponsor
- This is usually done on credit through advances from the sponsors
- Contract farming often introduces new technology and also enables farmers to learn new skills.
- Farmers price risk often reduced as many contracts specify price in advance.
- Lower transaction costs, assured markets, and better allocation of risks.
- Contract farming can open up new markets which would otherwise be unavailable to the small farmers.

### For Sponsors

- Working with small farmers overcome land constraints.
- Production is more reliable than open-market purchases and sponsoring company faces less risk by not being responsible for production.
- More consistent quality can be obtained than if purchases were made on the open market.

## Limitations of Contract Farming

There are various practical problems that emerge in contract farming that can result in losses to both farmers and firms.

### For Farmers

- In negotiating contracts, small-scale producers are in a weak position, lacking market power and information on patterns of supply, demand and prices.
- Sponsoring company may be unreliable or exploit a monopoly position.
- The staff of sponsoring organizations may be corrupt.

## For Sponsors

- ✰ Poor management and lack of consultation with farmers may lead to farmer discontent.
- ✰ Farmer may sell outside the contract.
- ✰ Farmers may divert inputs supplied on credit to other purposes, thereby reducing yields.

## Conclusion

Contract farming creates link farmers to a firm/processor. The firm offers technical assistance, delivers inputs on credit, and reduces market risk, solving a number of constraints that limit farm productivity and income. On the other hand, the farmer produces the farm products and agreed to sale it to the processor at predetermined price. Thus, contract farming should be considered an institution that has a positive effect on farmers. Wider use of this approach may allow contract farming to expand into new areas and commodities, helping to address some of the constraints faced by small farmers in developing countries. Gaps in the current knowledge of contract farming could be addressed by additional research.

## REFERENCES

Birthal, P.S. and Jha, A.K. (2005). Economic losses due to various constraints in dairy production in India. *Indian Journal of Animal Sciences*, 75: 1476-1480.

Birthal, P.S., Taneja, V.K. and Thorpe, W. (2006). Smallholder Livestock Production in India: Opportunities and Challenges. National Centre for Agricultural Economics and Policy Research, New Delhi, India and International Livestock Research Institute, Nairobi, Kenya.

Economic Survey 2017-18 Volume II. Government of India Ministry of Finance Department of Economic Affairs Economic Division January, 2018.

IGFRI. (2013). Vision 2050. ICAR-Indian Grassland and Fodder Research Institute, Gwalior Road, Jhansi.

Chapter 6

# Role of Herbal Nutraceuticals in Heath and Productivity of Livestock

*Y.P. Sahni, Kamal Kishor and R.P. Singh*

*Nanaji Deshmukh Veterinary Science University, Jabalpur, Madhya Pradesh*

Nutraceutical is a term coined in 1989 by Stephen DeFelice. It is defined as a food or parts of food that provide medical or health benefits, including the prevention and treatment of disease. Nutraceuticals may range from isolated nutrients, herbal products, dietary supplements, and diets to genetically engineered designer foods, and processed products such as cereals, soups, and beverages. A nutraceutical is any non-toxic food extract supplement that has scientifically proven health benefits for both the treatment and prevention of disease. Nutraceuticals also refer to natural functional/medical foods or bioactive phytochemicals that have health-promoting, disease preventing or medicinal properties. These nutraceuticals in general contain vitamins, lipids, proteins, carbohydrates, minerals, or other necessary nutrients. These nutraceuticals are used in nutritional therapy based upon their chemical structures and biological functions. Nutraceuticals are found in a mosaic of products emerging from the food industry, the commercial herbal, dietary supplement pharmaceutical industry and the newly merged pharmaceutical/agri-business/ nutrition conglomerates.

The goal of achieving an optimal or maximal state of nutrition and health is becoming an increasing challenge with the introduction of many nutraceuticas. Plant biotechnologists have put lots of effort to engineer plants and crops in order to improve their nutritional value to maintain a healthy human body. It has been proved that any excess intake of any nutrient may not benefit or even can be harmful to health. Already there are many plant biotechnological products currently, which are patented for their medicinal values. Products marketed as functional foods and nutraceuticals are highly variable and are often dependent upon historical if not local allegiances. Nutraceuticals are marketed in concentrated forms as pills, capsules, powders and tinctures either as a single substance or as combination preparations (Prabu *et al.,* 2012).

## Classification of Nutraceuticals

### Nutrients

The substances with established nutritional functions, such as vitamins, minerals, amino acids and fatty acids.

### Herbals

Herbs or botanical products as concentrates or extracts.

### Dietary Supplements

Individual compounds used in the therapy or prevention of deficiencies or when constant supply of a nutrient is required or when a missing enzyme is replaced.

### Potential Nutraceuticals

A potential nutraceutical is one that holds a promise of a particular health or medical benefit.

### Established Nutraceuticals

When sufficient clinical data of potential nutraceuticals is obtained on its health and medical benefits.

## Nutraceuticals as Therapeutic Agents

### Digestive Tonic and Growth Promoter

Supplementation of certain herbs that have property to modulate the rumen function may be supplementated to animals for efficient cellulose breakdown and digestion, maintenance of normal ruminoreticular functon, intestinal movement, optimum utilization and absorption of nutrients, thus improving feed conversion ratio, productivity and body weight gain in animals. Ruchamax is a potent herbal formulation, which contains 28 different herbs and some minerals. The ingredients of Ruchamax include *Allium sativum, Azadirachta indica, Calotrophis orocera, Centratherum anthelmenticum, Commiphora mukul, Eclipta elba, Embelica ribes, Picorrhiza kurora, Zinziber officinale* and *Piper longum etc.* It is used as an appetizer, restorative, stomachic, digestive tonic and growth promoter product (Kolte *et al.,* 2009).

## Gut Enhancer

Phytogenic substances from certain herbs *viz. Aegle marmelos, Plantago ovata, Acacia catechu, Corriandrum sativum,* many more herbs and their extracts have also been shown to improve gut microflora and to exert pharmacologic actions within the digestive tract, as evidenced by their gut function modulating efficacy (Satyavati, and Gupta, 1987). In the intestine, bacteria considered beneficial to the gut, including lactic acid forming bacteria like *Lactobacillus* spp, prevent proliferation of pathogens, such as *Salmonella* spp., through competitive exclusion for nutrients

## Feed Efficiency Intensifier

The addition of certain herbs *viz. Woodfordia fruticosa, Zingiber officinale, Allium sativum, Trigonella foenum graecum etc.* to poultry and pig ration is known to improve feed efficiency (Satyavati and Gupta, 1987). Increased palatability of the diets associated with the addition of phytogenies may be due to their anti-oxidative effects.

## Anti-oxidant, Immunomodulator and Antistressor

Herbs namely *Mangifera indica, Echinacea purpurea, Phyllanthus emblica, Uncaria tomentosa, Withania somnifera, Ocimum sanctum, Tinospora cordifolia, Asparagus racemosus* and many more are scientifically validated to possess antistressor, immunostimulant or immunomodulant and adaptogenic properties.

## Hepatic Stimulant

The herbal ingredients such as *Andrographis paniculata, Eclipta alba, Picrorhiza kurroa, Phyllanthus niruri, Tephrosia purpurea, Tinospora cardifolia and Boerhavia diffusa* (Superliv concentrate premix and Liquid) have been proved to improve feed conversion efficiency, body weight gain and reduce mortality in poultry and swine; owing to their Hepato-protective activity.

## Natural Methionine

Poultry feeding is one of the most important areas, since feed alone accounts for about 65-70 per cent cost of the total poultry enterprise. Protein synthesis in chickens is required at a very rapid pace for fast growing broilers and prolific layers. Methionine is required in free as well as conjugated form to perform various metabolic functions. It assists in the breakdown of fats and thereby prevents the build-up of fat in liver and arteries, as well as assisting the digestive system and removing heavy metals from the body since it can be converted to cysteine, which is a precursor to glutathione, which is of prime importance in detoxifying the liver (Ramarao *et al.,* 2003).

## Antimicrobial

Plants namely *Trichyspermum ammi, Cinamonum camphora, Mentha piperita, Oregano* and *thyme* are among those which have received a great deal of interest. These plants contain the monoterpenes carvacrol and thymol, respectively, and have demonstrated high efficacy *in vitro* against several pathogens found in the intestinal tract. This suggests that phytogenic feed additives may be suitable replacements for in- feed antibiotics to improve health and growth performance.

### Hypotensive

The consumption of flax seed may lower blood pressures lightly. The beneficial potential of ax seed to reduce blood pressure, especially diastolic blood pressure (DBP) may be greater when it is consumed as a whole seed and for duration of less than12 week. Flaxseed contains ω-3 fatty acids, lignans, and fiber that together may provide benefits to patients with cardiovascular disease. Animal work identified that patients with peripheral artery disease may particularly benefit from dietary supplementation with flaxseed. Circulating α-linolenic acid levels correlated with systolic blood pressure (SBP) and DBP, and lignan levels correlated with changes in DBP. Flaxseed is proven to be effective, it has many advantages as an anti-hypertensive treatment option for patients.

### Hypocholesteremic

Garlic (*Allium sativum*), Dhania (*Coriandrum sativum*), Arjun (*Terminalia arjuna*) *and Amla* (*Emblica officinalis*) *etc.* are known to reduces total cholesterol to a modest extent, without appreciable LDL lowering or HDL elevation. The essential oil fraction of garlic comprises 60 per cent of diallyl disulphide (DADS) which have hypocholesterolemic activity. The major sulfur-containing compounds in intact garlic are γ-glutamyl-S-allyl-l-cysteines and S-allyl-l-cysteine sulfoxides (alliin). Both are abundant as sulfur compounds, and alliin is the primary odorless, sulfur-containing amino acid, a precursor of allicin. Alliinase is the key enzyme that facilitates the transformation of cysteine sulfoxides to thiosulfinates such as allicin. γ-Glutamyl- Sallyl-l-cysteines are converted into S-allylcysteines (SAC) through an enzymatic transformation with γ-glutamyltranspeptidase. Several clinical reports and meta- analyses have revealed the cholesterol lowering effects of garlic supplementation.

### Dermatological Conditions

There is early evidence that turmeric/curcumin products and supplements both oral and topical may provide therapeutic benefits for skin health.

## Mechanism of Action of Nutraceuticals

Evidences indicate that the mechanistic actions of natural compounds involve a wide array of biological processes, including activation of antioxidant defenses, signal transduction pathways, cell survival-associated gene expression, cell proliferation and differentiation and preservation of mitochondrial integrity. It appears that these properties play a crucial role in the protection against the pathologies of numerous age- related or chronic diseases. It is very imperative that the nutrients found in many foods, fruits and vegetables are responsible for the well documented health benefits (Bhowmik *et al.,* 2013).

The mechanism through which nutraceuticals prevent chronic diseases has not been fully elucidated. Many of these phytochemicals have been found to alter antioxidant defence of cells through the induction of DNA repair processes or enzymic antioxidant defence at the gene level. It has been suggested that they may also affect cell cycle progression, cell communication, hormone and growth factor signaling and apoptosis. Lycopene, a potent hypocholesterolemic agent found in tomato has been shown to prevent atherosclerosis by inhibiting LDL-C oxidation. Also, indole-3- carbinol, the most vital and important indole present in broccoli has been found to inhibit the Human Papilloma Virus (HPV) that may cause uterine cancer. This phytochemical acts by blocking the estrogen receptors specifically present in the breast cancer cells as well as down regulating CDK6, and up regulating p21 and p27 in prostate cancer cells. It brings about G1 cell-cycle arrest and apoptosis of breast and prostate cancer cells significantly and enhances the p 53 expression in cells treated with benzopyrene. It also depresses Akt, NF-kappaB, MAPK, and Bel-2 signaling pathways to an appreciably good extent (Olaiya *et al.,* 2016).

## Nutraceuticals in Research and Development

The greatest scientific need in nutraceuticals pertains to standardization of compounds and/or products, to carefully develop and execute clinical studies/trials to provide the basis for health claims for nutraceuticals that impact consumers as well as companies making strategic investments. Powerful market forces are fueling the interest in nutraceuticals (Pandey *et al.,* 2010). Research on nutraceuticals should be addressed:

- To test safety, purity and potency of products.
- To develop more effective and efficient means of producing ingredients for use in products.
- To develop testing methods for ensuring and verifying the consistency of the dosage of ingredients included in the company's products.
- To develop the new products either by combining existing ingredients used in nutritional supplements or identifying new ingredients that can be used in nutritional supplements.

## Market Trends

Nutraceutical is a new buzzword in Indian healthcare market. This promising term reflects lucrative market opportunities for domestic as well as international pharmaceutical and Nutraceutical companies. Nutraceuticals has a spectacular annual growth rate of 25 per cent in Indian healthcare market. It is estimated that, by end of 2007 global Nutraceutical market may cross USD 80 bn. The Indian nutraceutical market valued at \$ 1,480 million in 2011 could grow to \$ 2,731 million in 2016, a report said today. According to the report by business research and consulting firm Frost and Sullivan, functional foods will be the quickest growing category followed by dietary supplements until 2015. However, dietary supplements specifically herbal and dietetic supplements, will form the greatest opportunity areas for nutraceutical manufacturers, it added. Nutraceutical a portmanteau of the words 'nutrition' and 'pharmaceutical', is a food or food product that reportedly provides health and medical benefits, including the prevention and treatment of diseases. The report said that at present the dietary supplements were the largest category accounting for 64 per cent of the nutraceuticals market. This market is driven primarily by the pharmaceutical sector in the form of vitamin and mineral supplements, it added. As per the study the global nutraceutical market was estimated to be $ 149.5 billion in 2011 with US, Europe and Japan being the largest regional markets, accounting for nearly 93 per cent of the global nutraceutical demand (Bhowmik *et al.,* 2013).

## The Future of Nutraceuticals

Increasing awareness levels about fitness and health, spurred by media coverage are prompting the majority of people to lead healthier lifestyles, exercise more, and eat healthy. The expanding nutraceutical market indicates that end users are seeking minimally processed food with extra nutritional benefits and organoleptic value. This development, in turn, is propelling expansion in the nutraceutical markets globally. The emerging nutraceuticals industry seems destined to occupy the landscape in the new millennium. Its tremendous growth has implications for the food, pharmaceutical, healthcare, and agricultural industries. Many scientists believe that enzymes represent another exciting frontier in nutraceuticals. "Enzymes have been underemployed. They are going to be a hot area in the future." Fermentation technology using microbes to create new food products also represents potential. Global trends to healthy products cannot be reversed. Companies taking the lead by investing strategically in science, product development, marketing and consumer education will not go unrewarded (Radhika *et al.,* 2011).

## Conclusion

The nutraceutical industry is growing at a rate far exceeding expansion in the food and pharmaceutical industries. In tomorrow's market, the most successful nutraceutical players are likely to be those companies in which functional product are just a part of a broad line of goods satisfying both conventional and health value point. Future demand of nutraceutical depends on consumer perception of the relationship between diet and disease. the entire regulatory framework of dietary supplements in view of the role of nutraceuticals is deemed necessary to first give credit to their different purposes and definition, and second, to assess their septic role in the prevention and treatment of pathological conditions, supporting their potential medical use in prevention and therapy only when proven by sound scientific and clinical data. The specificity of nutraceuticals would need a premarket approval system substantiated by scientific data (*in vivo* clinical trials) showing their complete safety and efficacy profile. The regulatory approach could be based on the one adopted for drugs, which is stricter and more complex. The likelihood of this occurring in the foreseeable future is unfortunately quite low. However, some measures could result in improvements of the existing situation. It may be reasonable for national competent authorities to ask manufacturers to provide data on the safety, efficacy and mechanism of action supporting any claims contained on the labels of their products, especially when the term nutraceutical is used. Strict guidelines would be needed and shared at international level to ensure that proper information is used to substantiate any health claims on the product label and detailed in the recommendation/safety guidelines, which should be included in the packaged products.

## REFERENCES

Bhowmik, D., Gopinath, H., Kumar, B.P., Duraivel, S. and Kumar, K.P.S. (2013). Nutraceutical- A bright scope and opportunity of Indian healthcare market. *"The Pharma Innovation" Journal*, **1**(11).

Kolte, A.Y., Maini, S., Ravikanth, K. and Rekhe, D.S. (2009). Role of polyherbal formulation in modulating rumen biochemical and growth performance parameters in calves. *Internet Journal of Veterinary Medicine*, **6**(2).

Olaiya, C.O., Soetan, K.O. and Esan, A.M. (2016). The role of nutraceuticals, functional food and value added food products in the prevention and treatment of chronic disease. *African Journal of Food Science*, **10**(10): 185-193.

Pandey, M., Verma R.K. and Saraf, S.A. (2010). Nutraceuticals: new era of medicine and health. *Asian Journal of Pharmaceutical and Clinical Research*, **3**(1): 0974-2441.

Prabu, S.L., Suriyaprakash, T.N.K., Kumar, C.D. and Kumar, S.S. (2012). Nutraceuticals and their medicinal importance. *International Journal of Health and Allied Sciences*, **1**(2).

Radhika, P.R., Singh, R.B.M. and Sivakumar, T. (2011). Nutraceuticals: An area of tremendous scope. *International Journal of Research in Ayurveda and Pharmacy*, **2**(2): 410-415.

Rama Rao, S.V., Panda, A.K., Raju, M.V.L.N., Shyamsunder R.G. and Praharaj, N.K. (2003). Requirement of calcium for commercial broiler and white leghorn layers at low dietary phosphorus levels. *Animal Feed Science Technology*, **106**: 199-208.

Satyavati, G.V. and Gupta, A.K. (1987). Medicinal plant of India. Indian Council of Medical Research, 2: 541.

## Chapter 7

# Nutritional Strategies to Improve Reproductive Efficiency of Dairy Animals in Rural Areas

*S.N. Shukla*

*Department of Animal Reproduction Gynaecology and Obstetrics, College of Veterinary Science and Animal Husbandry, Nanaji Deshmukh Veterinary Science University, Jabalpur, Madhya Pradesh*

Reproductive efficiency is a major component of economic success in dairy herds. Unfortunately, fertility in dairy cows involves extremely complex biological events that are influenced by a multitude of environmental and biological factors, as well as the genetic makeup of the dairy cow. Over recent decades, genetic improvement and better management practices have dramatically increased milk production but, at the same time it become difficult to manage fertility and conception rate of the farm animals. Managing optimum productivity of dairy animals in terms of quality milk production and efficient breeding plays a vital role in profitable dairy farming. Poor nutrition delays puberty, reduces conception rate and increases pregnancy losses in heifers. It has been seen that critical age-to-weight ratio which must be reached before heifers attain puberty. Feeding concentrates to zebu cows advanced puberty and first conception by 4 to 18 months.

Nutrition is one of the most important factors in their performance, health and welfare. Many nutrients are utilized by the body for milk production, and increased nutrient demands for production can negatively impact reproduction in dairy cows. High-yielding cows require special nutritional care, especially during periods of production stress *i.e.* during lactation or in advanced pregnancy. Meeting the nutritional needs of the high-yielding cow for optimum production and reproduction is a challenge for dairy producers. An adequately nourished cow will be healthy and capable of managing the stresses associated with high milk production.

The negative energy balance during post-partal critical period causes problems in reproduction, as energy status is linked with delayed ovulation. Energy deprivation reduces the frequency of LH pulses, thereby impairing follicle maturation and ovulation. Furthermore, undernutrition inhibits estrous behavior partly because of reduced estrogen receptor-alpha abundance in the brain. Balance diet consisting of energy and protein feed ingredients, in addition to many trace elements and vitamins, play important roles in milk production and reproduction. It is not only the quantities of energy and protein source, but also their quality that plays a vital role for optimum production and reproduction.

## Additional Supplementation of Energy

In lactating dairy cows especially during peak milk yield (four to eight weeks postpartum) the dry matter intake does not increase proportionately to meet energy requirements until 10-14 weeks postpartum. Consequently, high-yielding cows experience some degree of negative energy balance during the early postpartum period. High-yielding cows have a gap between energy supply and demand. To fulfil the higher energy need for milk production, animals utilize body reserves resulting in impaired health and frequent metabolic disorders. Energy is the major nutrient required by adult cow; and inadequate energy intake has a detrimental impact on milk yield and reproduction. Cows under negative energy balance have extended periods of anovulation. Postpartum anestrus, as well as infertility, is magnified by losses of body condition during the early postpartum period.

## Strategies to Increase Energy Intake

The extent and duration of postpartum negative energy balance is influenced by genetic potentiality for milk production, dietary energy density and dry matter intake. Nutritional management strategies can be employed to minimize the extent and duration of negative energy balance. In view of the fact that dry matter intake during the early lactation period goes down, increasing energy density of the ration is the only available option to improve energy intake, which can be achieved through supplementation of grains or fat. Diets containing high levels of grain may cause metabolic disturbances, such as rumen acidosis, and may ultimately result in low milk and milk fat production. To avoid these problems, fat can be added to increase the energy density of the diet. Fat supplementation also has other potential benefits, such as increased absorption of fat-soluble nutrients and reduced dustiness of feed. In addition, feeding fat to dairy cows generally improves fertility.

## Dietary Supplementation with Fat

Fat supplementation may improve fertility. Good body condition at calving is very important to minimize negative energy balance. At the time of dry-off, aim for a body condition score (BCS) of at least 3.0 and at calving, 3.5 to 4.0, but be cautious not to over-condition. Obese cows (BCS >4.0) tend to have a higher incidence of calving difficulty, retained placenta and possibly compromised health and reproductive parameters. During the post calving period, increase the energy intake (by feeding higher levels of bypass fat) so that a positive energy balance is achieved with minimum loss of body condition.

From what is currently known, fat supplementation exerts beneficial effects on reproduction. Long chain polyunsaturated fatty acids such as linoleic acid are known to stimulate reproductive function. Other fatty acids that are known to influence reproductive function are linolenic acid, eicosapentaenoic acid and docosahexaenoic acid. Fat supplements that have improved fertility of lactating dairy cows include fish meal, tallow and calcium soaps of palm oil. A recently it is reported significantly higher (89 per cent) non return rates to first insemination in dairy cows that were fed formaldehyde- treated flaxseed. Treating oil seeds with formaldehyde is known to protect fatty acids from the rumen environment, thereby allowing an increased delivery of fatty acids in a protected form to the lower gut.

How does fat influence reproduction? Firstly, fat supplementation increases the overall number of ovarian follicles and size of the dominant follicle. Secondly, an increase in plasma cholesterol often occurs following dietary fat supplementation. Since cholesterol is a precursor for progesterone (PG), the increased availability of cholesterol may contribute to an increasedconcentration of progesterone in plasma. The third mechanism by which dietary fats may enhance reproductive efficiency is via a reduction in endometrial PG secretion.

## Dietary Supplementation of Protein

It is very essential for growth, maintenance and production. Dairy cows require essential amino acids that must be absorbed from the small intestine. Ruminants obtain amino acids from two sources – microbial proteins and bypass protein, or rumen undegraded protein. A high intake of rumen degradable protein increases concentrations of urea nitrogen in plasma and vaginal mucus resulting in lowered fertility. Sperm viability and embryo development is reportedly affected by the presence of excessive urea in the reproductive tract of cows. To reduce the possibility of these negative effects, do not supply rumen degradable proteins in excess of the needs of the cow.

## Minerals and Vitamins

The lack of minerals (Ca, P, Zn, Cu, Mn *etc.*) is related to various reproductive problems in livestock. Phosphorus deficiency causes infertility by affecting normal physiological functioning of reproductive organs. It also decreases total dry matter intake resulting in to lower energy supply and hampering weight gain especially in stress conditions. Low concentration of serum Ca, Mg, and Fe was recorded in repeat breeder as compared to normal cows. The serum concentration of Ca, P, Cu and Zn was reported to be low in anoestrous cows. The increase chance of non infectious endometritis especially during low Ca:P ratio in the diets of animals. Chromium is an essential element that is required for the efficient utilisation of dietary energy. Glucose, produced from carbohydrates, is one of the major sources of energy. Insulin takes major part in the glucose metabolism. Chromium acts biologically as a component of glucose tolerance factor, which enhances tissue sensitivity to insulin and glucose utilization. It improves reproductive performance, cell-mediated and humoral-immune responses. Chromium helps reduce the effect of physiological stress. Area specific mineral mixture may be advised as per deficiency of the same in the animals.

**Table 7.1. Summary of Important Micronutrients Affecting Animal Reproduction**

| *Micronutrient* | *Function* | *Consequence-deficiency* |
|---|---|---|
| Vitamin A | Maintain the integrity of the reproductive tract and favors the reproductive process in females and males. | Stops puberty in both females and males; predisposes to low rates of fertilization and embryo mortality, as well as placental retention and reduces male sexual desire. |
| Vitamin E | It promotes and maintains the reproductive life. | Placental retention and predisposes males to malformations and low sperm count in the ejaculate. |
| Selenium | It acts as cofactor cell peroxidase enzyme system responsible for the intra and extra glutathione oxidation of the cell membrane of the cells that make up the reproductive tract. | Predisposes to low fertility; placental retention and disposition to ovarian cysts; in males, reduced sperm motility and concentration. |
| Copper | It promotes hormonal physiology and prostaglandin synthesis. | Predisposition to low fertility; estrous cycle disorders, embryonic and fetal death; abortions and placenta retention. |
| Zinc | It promotes the function of several metabolic enzymes and hormone function in males and females. | Predisposition to low fertility, prolificacy and retained placenta; in males, spermatogenesis and harms the development of secondary sexual organs. |
| Chromium | Chromium is an essential element that is required for the efficient utilisation of dietary energy. Glucose, produced from carbohydrates, is one of the major sources of energy. Insulin takes major part in the glucose metabolism. Chromium acts biologically as a component of glucose tolerance factor, which enhances tissue sensitivity to insulin and glucose utilization. | It improves reproductive performance, cell- mediated and humoral-immune responses. Chromium helps reduce the effect of physiological stress. |

Vitamin deficiency is one of the important causes of reproductive failure in cattle and buffaloes causing delayed onset of puberty, abortion and abnormal calf birth. The major vitamins affecting reproduction are Vitamine A, E, D and β-carotene. In dairy cows vit. A deficiency is responsible for premature birth, abortion and birth of blind calves. Vitamin-A plays an important role in animal reproduction. The deficiency of vitamin-A in male animals delays sexual maturity, causing poor sex drive, abnormal spermatogenesis and impotentia. In heifer and milking cows the negative effect of β-carotene deficiency on fertility was recorded which is not related to vitamin-A.

It brief it is required to adopt at least minimum strategic feeding for better reproductive performance and thus production in dairy animals which includes green forage supplementation of concentrate, oilseed meals and fat, and minerals especially area specific mineral mixture. The feeding standards can be modified as per the production potential and genetic makeup of animals to minimize health and reproductive problems.

Chapter 8

# Indian Breed Cow Milk: A2 Milk Powerhouse of Health

*S.K. Joshi, M.S. Thakur, Vaishali Khare, R.K. Vandre and Akhilesh Pandey*

*Department of Animal Genetics and Breeding, College of Veterinary Science and Animal Husbandry, Nanaji Deshmukh Veterinary Science University, Jabalpur, Madhya Pradesh*

According to Hindu mythology and sayings of sages the Kamadhenu is the mother of all cows. Since thousands of years, we worship cow as ¯Kamadhenu, the God who fulfills our desires. Cows are venerated as the earthly embodiment of Kamadhenu. The Indian breeds of cows are a crucial part of the country's ecological heritage. In thse past, these breeds were developed in different parts of the subcontinent by selecting the best animals for their preferred traits such as milking capacity, draught power, feeding requirements, capacity to adapt to local weather, immunity *etc.* The purity of such breeds was maintained with great discipline and wisdom in each breeding tract.

However, since the sixties, in a order to increase the milk production of Indian breeds (Bos indicus) the Indian Government has resorted to ¯cross-breeding by using foreign bulls and semen (Bos Taurus). This definitely improved milk production but also lead to gradual extinction of our low-maintenance, superior enduring variety of native breed of cows. Most recently the concept of A1 and A2 milk realized again the superiority and importance of our indigenous cattle breeds.

Interest in the distinction between A1 and A2 milk began in the early 1990s via epidemiological research and animal studies initially conducted by scientists in New Zealand, which found correlations between the prevalence of milk with A1 beta- casein proteins in some countries and the prevalence of various chronic diseases. The research generated interest in the media, as well as among the scientific community and entrepreneurs.

## The Difference Between A1 and A2 Milk

Cows' milk is about 87 per cent water and 13 per cent solids, the solids being a combination of fat, carbohydrates in the form of lactose, minerals, and protein. The protein component in milk is made up of up to 80 per cent casein (Pehrsson *et al.,* 2000,); in turn about 30-35 per cent of the casein (equivalent to two teaspoons in a litre of milk) is beta-casein, of which there are several varieties, determined by the genes of the cow. The most common of these variants are A1 and A2 (named for the order in which they were identified by scientists), with the sole difference between the two being one of the 209 amino acids that make up the beta-casein proteins: a proline occurs at position 67 in the chain of amino acids that make up the A2 beta-casein, while in A1 beta-casein a histidine occurs at that position. Studies in cells found that digestive enzymes that cut up proteins interact with beta-casein precisely at that location, so that A1 and A2 beta- casein proteins are processed differently. A seven-aminoacid peptide, beta- casomorphin-7, (BCM-7) can be cut away from the A1-beta-casein protein by those enzymes, but the enzymes cannot cut the A2 protein at that location, so BCM-7 is not formed from A2 proteins.

Around 5,000 years ago, a mutation occurred in this proline amino acid, converting it to histidine. Cows that have this mutated beta casein protein are called A1 cows. The A1 gene mutation began hundreds of years ago from Holstein cow breed that was then passed onto other breeds.The percentage of the A1 and A2 beta-casein protein varies between herds of cattle, and also between countries and provinces. While African and Asian cattle continue to produce only A2 beta-casein, the A1 version of the protein is common among cattle in the western world. The A1 beta-casein type is the most common type found in cow's milk in Europe (excluding France), the USA, Australia and New Zealand. On average, more than 70 per cent of Guernsey cows produce milk with predominantly A2 protein, while among Holsteins and Ayrshires between 46 and 70 per cent produce A1 milk.

- ✰ **A1 beta-casein** comes from the most common cow breed that originated in Australia, United States, and Northern Europe. This includes Holstein, Friesian, Ayrshire, and British Shorthorn cow breeds that contains A1 beta-casein.
- ✰ **A2 beta-casein** is protein found in milk produced by all of the Indian cow breeds and some of exotic breeds like the Jersey, Charolais, Guernsey, and Limousin. Milk produced by other mammals such as those from human, goat, and sheep is also contains A2 beta-casein.

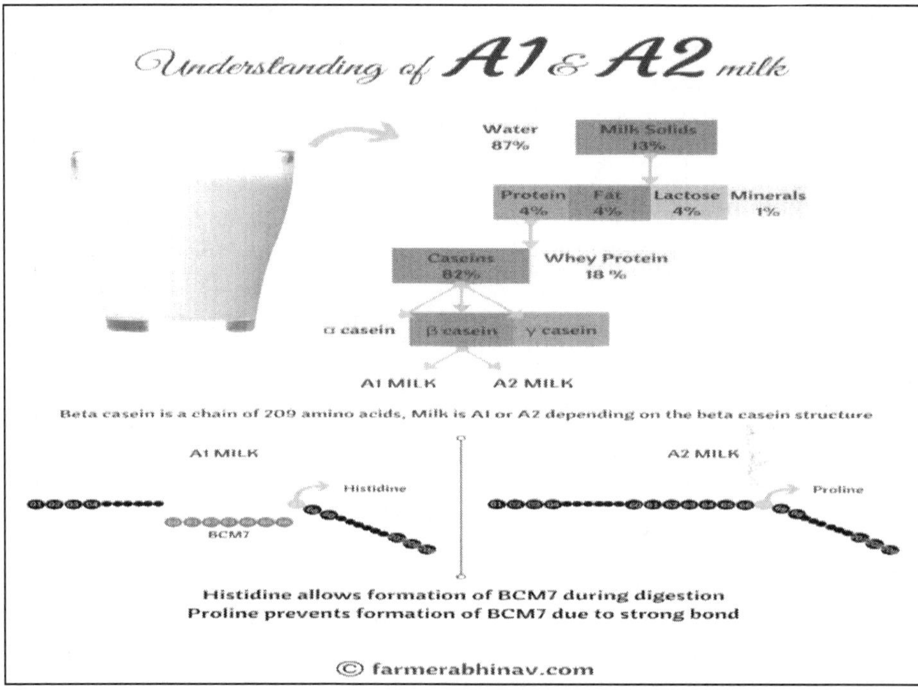


☆ Proline has a strong bond to a small protein called BCM7 and therefore stops the BCM7 from getting into milk. So essentially, no BCM7 is found in the urine, blood or gastro-intestinal tracts of the original A2 cows. Histidine, the mutated protein, does not have a strong bond to hold on to BCM7. Hence, on consumption of the A1 milk, this protein BCM7 gets into the gastro-intestinal tract of animals and humans (Truswell, 2005).

## What is BCM7?

**BCM7 (Beta-casomorphin-7)**, an opioid peptide in A1 beta-casein is produced as a result of the breaking off of histidine in the number 67 amino acid chain during digestion. BCM7 found in A1 milk is known to have opioid or narcotic side effects and is identified to be the culprit of lactose intolerance in 1 out 4 Americans.The absorption of BCM7 into the bloodstream leads to the high incidence of autism, schizophrenia, and other neurological disorders (Wasilewska *et al.,* 2011).

## A1/A2 Milk in Relation to Calcium : Magnesium Ratio

With the increasing intake of dairy products, the consumption of other essential nutrients such as zinc, vitamin A, magnesium, folate, and riboflavin are also increasing. However, we are able to get only about 700 mg of calcium per day, which comes primarily from dairy products. This amount is against the recommended amount of 1,000–1,500 mg. Most other food sources contain low concentrations of calcium. Calcium content of milk may reduce the risk of osteoporosis and colon cancer and including milk in the diet may promote weight loss. The ideal calcium to magnesium ratio for the human body should be 2:1. The A1 milk's ratio is 10:1. By relying on A1 cow's milk for calcium, we will have magnesium deficiency and imbalance, but A2 milk does not cause such imbalances. Magnesium relaxes us, helps improve digestion, is anti-inflammatory in action, involved in nerve and muscle function, de-toxifier, increases alkalinity of the blood and flexibility of the tissues. Magnesium is required for the body to produce and store energy. Without magnesium there is no energy, no movement, no life. So, A1 milk will lower magnesium levels whereas A2 milk does not (Weinberg *et al.,* 2004).

## Health Hazards of A1 Milk Type 1 Diabetes Mellitus

Type 1 Diabetes Mellitus is an autoimmune disease that typically develops in children. According to a 1992 observational study by Laugesen and Elliott in 2003, there was low incidence of diabetes mellitus type 1 among infants who were breastfed in the Polynesian Islands as opposed to Polynesian infants in Auckland that were supplied with commercial milk formulations containing A1 beta-casein.

### Heart Diseases

According to New Zealand research conducted by CNS McLachlan, the regular intake of common milk containing A1 beta-casein inspires the development of coronary heart disease (Laugesen and Elliott, 2003).

### Sudden Infant Death Syndrome (SIDS)

The most common cause of death in infants less than one year of age is identified to be Sudden Infant Death Syndrome or SIDS. It is unexpected infant death without clear or visible cause (28).

Some researchers hypothesized that BCM-7 from A1 beta-casein may be the culprit in some cases of SIDs (Wasilewska *et al.,* 2011).

### Autism

Autism is a developmental disorder characterized by disabilities including problems with social interaction, communication, and repetitive behaviors. It was theorized that BCM-7 plays a crucial role in the development of autism in children. In a study conducted by Russian researchers, high amounts of BCM-7 were found in the urine of infants with autism that were fed with milk formula. Over time, there were infants that showed the ability to metabolize BCM-7 at a fast rate, whilst there are those who showcased inability to process and excrete BCM-7 and other peptides altogether (Cass *et al.,* 2008).

### Lactose Intolerance

Based on studies, 1 in 4 Americans suffer from lactose intolerance, the inability if the digestive system to process milk resulting in the development of unpleasant symptoms such as stomach upsets, diarrhea, flatulence, and bloating to name a few. A1 and A2 milk feature the same lactose concentrations. The makers of A2 milk contend that lactose is not the real suspect for the development of lactose intolerance, but a mutation caused by A1 beta-casein, a compound found in store-brought milk and dairy products (Pelto *et al.,* 1999).

## Scientific Evidence for A1 Milk Health Effects

The first arguments in favour of A2 milk have been made basis two studies which correlated the average per capita consumption of A1 beta-casein and the incidence of certain diseases in various countries. One of the studies was published by Laugesen and Elliott, 2003 showing incidence of type 1 diabetese and consumption of A1 beta casein and the other study by MacLachlan 2001 showing incidence of heart disease death rate and consumption of A1 beta casein. The graphs showing the correlation in these studies are shown below:

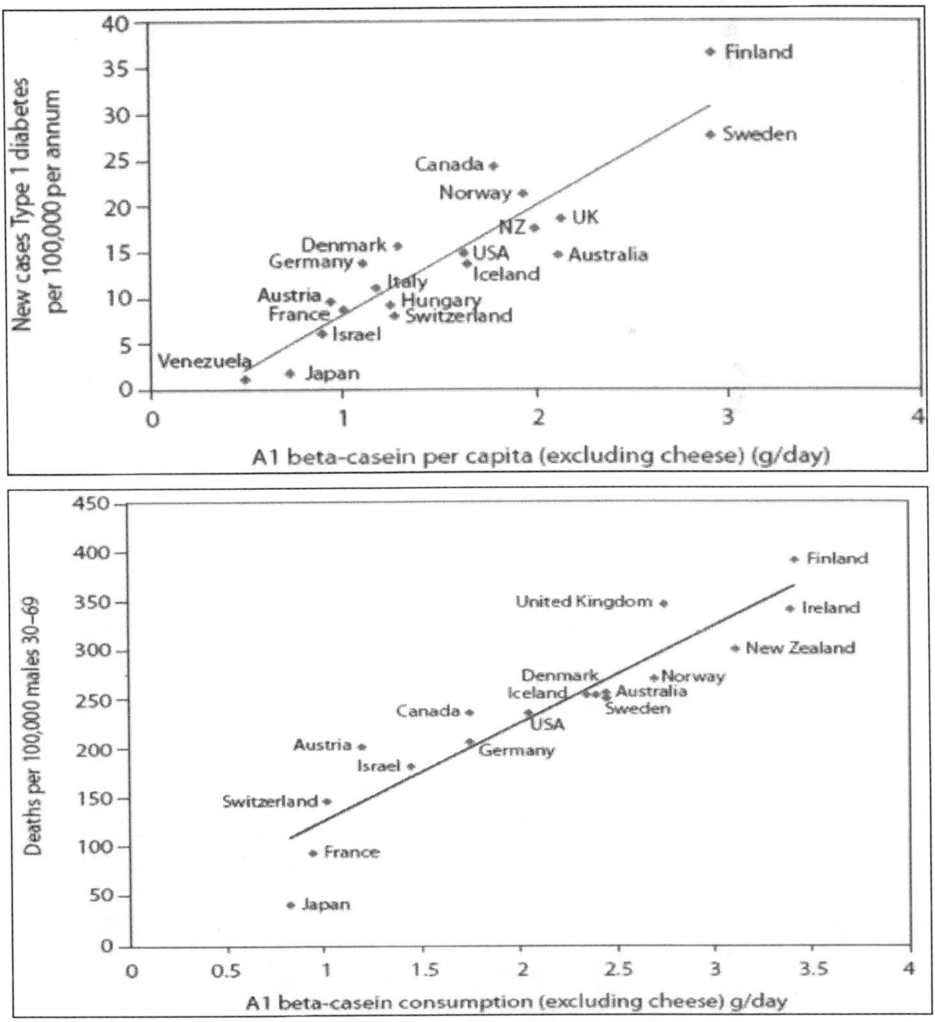


**Type 1 Diabetes and A1 Beta-casein Consumption.**

## Status of Milk Protein Variants in Cattle

Researches conducted on indigenous cows (Zebu type), buffaloes and exotic cows (Taurine type) have revealed that A1 allele is more frequent in exotic cattle (A1 milk) while Indian native dairy cows and buffaloes have only A2 allele and hence are a source for safe milk i.e A2 milk. Mishra *et al.* (2009) investigated frequency of beta casein variants among 618 animals of 15 zebu cattle breeds and 213 buffaloes of 8 river buffalo breeds. The study revealed predominance of A2 variants (98.7 per cent) in zebu cattle while river buffalo indicated only A2 milk type.

## Conclusion

Milk from dairy cows is providing a high quality source of protein and an essential micronutrients like energy, calcium, magnesium and phosphorus to human beings since long time (Bell *et al.,* 2006). The Food and Agriculture Organisation (FAO) (2012) has reported increase in many chronic diseases arising out of milk. These diseases if studied thoroughly can be alleviated by improving the health benefiting milk components. The β-casein composition of the protein fraction has become of special interest recently because of a possible relationship between β-casein genotype and the health of population of consumers. Genetic variants in bovine β-casein gene (A1 and B) release a bioactive peptide, β-casomorphin-7(BCM-7) upon digestion, responsible for many human disorders like Type 1 diabetes, autism, schizophrenia and heart diseases but A2 milk does not cause such type of illnesses (Mishra *et al.,* 2009). Infants may absorb β-CM-7 due to an immature gastrointestinal tract. Adults, on the other hand, appear to reap the biological activity locally on the intestinal brush boarder. B-CM-7 can potentially affect numerous opioid receptors in the nervous, endocrine, and immune systems. Realizing the severe ill effects of A1 milk the breeding strategies should be directed to conserve our indigenous breeds which provide the superior A1 milk.

## REFERENCES

Cass, H., Gringras, P., March, J., McKendrick, I., O'Hare, A.E., Owen, L., Pollin, C.(2008). Absence of urinary opioid peptides in children with autism. *Arch Dis Child.* **293**(9): 745-50.

Laugesen, M, Elliott, R. (2003).Ischaemic heart disease, type 1 diabetes, and cow milk A1 beta-casein. *N Z Med J.,* p. 116.

McLachlan, C.N. (2001). beta-casein A1, ischaemic heart disease mortality, and other illnesses Med Hypotheses. **56**(2): 262-72.

Mishra, B.P., Mukesh, M., Prakash, B., Sodhi, M., Kapila, R., kishore, A., Kataria, R.S., Joshi, B. K., Rasool, T.J.and Bujarbaruah, K.M. (2009) Status of milk protein, β-casein variants among Indian milch animals. *Indian Journal of Animal Sciences* **79** (7), 722–725.

Pehrsson, P.R., Haytowitz, D.B.; Holden, J.M.; Perry, C.R.; Beckler, D.G. (2000). USDA's National Food and Nutrient Analysis Program: Food Sampling. *Journal of Food Composition and Analysis*, **13** (4): 379–389.

Pelto, L., Impivaara, O., Salminen, S., Poussa, T., Seppänen, R., Lilius, E.M.(1999).

Milk hypersensitivity in young adults. *Eur J Clin Nutr.* **53**(8): 620-624.

Truswell AS (2005). The A2 milk case: a critical review. *Eur J Clin Nutr.* **59**(5): 623- 31.

Wasilewska, J., Sienkiewicz-Sz³apka, E., KuŸbida, E., Jarmo³owska, B., Kaczmarski,

M. and Kostyra, E. (2011). The exogenous opioid peptides and DPPIV serum activity in infants with apnoea expressed as apparent life threatening events (ALTE). *Neuropeptides,* **45**(3): 189-95.

Weinberg, L.G., Berner, L.A. and Groves, J.E. (2004). Nutrient contribution of dairy foods in the United States, continuing survey of food intakes by individuals. *J. Am. Dietet. Assoc,* **104**: 895–902.

Chapter 9

# Application of Nutrigenomics Tools in Animal Feeding

*M.S. Thakur, Shrikant Joshi, R.K. Vandre, Vaishali Khare and Akhilesh Pandey*

*Department of Animal Genetics and Breeding, College of Veterinary Science and Animal Husbandry, Nanaji Deshmukh Veterinary Science University, Jabalpur, Madhya Pradesh*

## Introduction

The human genome project has started the new era of biology. The completion of this brought many marked breakthroughs in science and technology. This new era based on functional genomics is the direct result of the massive accumulation of information that is resulting from studies of a variety of animal, plant, and microbial genomes. Applications of molecular technology provide new ways to evaluate reproductive potential and the basic physiological mechanisms that limit reproductive performance. The performance traits of livestock are thought to be affected by genotype (heritable) and environment (non-heritable). Nutrition is among the greatest environmental determinants. Genes are turned on and off according to metabolic signals that the nucleus receives from internal factors like hormones and external factors like nutrients. Nutrigenomics is emerging in the area of livestock to develop feeds that can be matched to genotypes of animals for a better production and health. Diet on its own or by interaction with other environmental factors can cause epigenetic changes that may turn certain genes on or off. Nutrigenomics has great emphasis due to its great potentiality to select animals for feed conversion efficiency, production and quality improvement of products. It deciphers how food ingredients and nutrition affect gene expression, metabolic pathways and diet related disease development. Hence, Nutrigenomics makes clear that how gene interacts with nutrients and how DNA and genetic code affect the needs for certain nutrients and quantities which suggests the possibility to change the way we feed and manage livestock and poultry. The central role that nutrients play in governing the cell content of different proteins has been further investigated and a recognition of their role as regulators of gene transcription, nuclear RNA processing, *m*RNA stability and *m*RNA degradation has emerged.

The tools of molecular genetics are expected to have much more impact in the future. The interaction between diets and genes could be evaluated through DNA microarray techniques and quantitative real-time polymerase chain reaction (PCR). These profiling techniques are reported to allow examination of nutrient effects that was not possible in the past. Nutrigenomics is feasible to apply in livestock production but can only provide part of the solution in response to non genetic factors involved in livestock health and production.

Now days, in the developed country cereals are used for bio-fuel companies for production of biodiesel and ethanol (Schmidt, 2007). So that, the consumption of crops in farm animal is important to hold good revenue and this could be possible via nutrigenomics approach (Wang *et al.,* 2008). Application of this technique provides a new rapid test for evaluating nutrient induced physiological changes and efficient methods to evaluate interaction between nutrients for better production and health (Swanson *et al.,* 2003).

## Basic Principles of Nutrigenomics

The basic principles of nutrigenomics are:

- Substances contained in the food (micro- and macro-nutrients) can directly or indirectly affect the human genome through changes in its structure and gene expression.
- Under certain circumstances and in some individuals the diet can be an important risk factor for the development of the number of diseases.
- Some genes regulated by active substances in the diet probably play a crucial role in the onset, incidence, progression and severity of the disease.
- The degree to which diet influences the balance between health and disease may depend on individual's genetic makeup.
- Nutritional intervention is based on the knowledge of individual's nutritional status and needs as well as genotype (individualized nutrition) and can be used for prevention, mitigation or healing the chronic diseases.

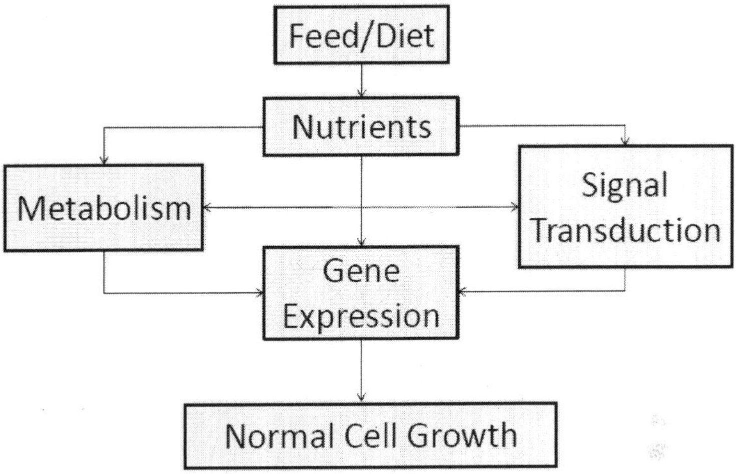


## Effect of Diet on Gene Expression and Metabolism in Livestock Species

Food derived from animals is an important source of nutrients in diets and the demand for high-quality meat and dairy products will rise over the next 20 years, accompanied by more stringent quality assurance requirements. Nutrigenomic approaches offer the potential to develop enhanced systems that overcome some of the existing limitations of production (Andersen *et al.,* 2005). Nutrigenomics offers the potential to improve animal production enterprises through major health and productivity gains. Animal products are a significant source of high-quality protein, calcium and iron, but have also been identified as a major source of excessive saturated fat intakes. Animal derived food contributes around 30 per cent of the total energy input, over 50 per cent of which is derived from fat.

Nutritional genomics has many prospects for applications in animal production. Animal scientists are already responding to the consumer demands for high standards of safety, nutritional value, texture and flavour, tenderness, water-holding capacity, colour and lipid content, lipid composition, oxidative stability and uniformity.

The new researches into molecular interactions of dietary nutrients have revealed that gene expression is altered by a number of dietary components such as proteins, carbohydrates, fatty acids, vitamins and minerals as well as phytochemicals (flavonoids, isothicyanates *etc.*). Most traits of interest for meat production have a multifactorial background, *i.e.*, meat attributes are due to interaction between the complex genetic background and the environment, with feeding being the most decisive factor in animal production. Feeding has a regulatory effect on biological processes in muscle, which is directly reflected in the quality of the meat, among other tissues. The knowledge of the complex interaction between the individual nutrients and their interaction on the genome of farm animals, which represent 30–40,000 genes within each species, is practically an unexplored area. The major reason for this is that the technical resources for such understanding have only become accessible within the past few years. The ongoing mapping of the genomes of the principal farm animals together with the progress within information technology and molecular biological techniques has accelerated this process (Andersen *et al.,* 2005 and Benitez *et al.,* 2017).

## Tools of Nutrigenomics

Transcriptomics, Proteomics and Metabolomics are the three crucial stages of nutrigenomics. Tools of transcriptomics (microarray technologies) allowed new information concerning the physiological effect of dietary proteins; proteomics tools (two-dimensional electrophoresis) might be an important tool to explore the effect of individual amino acid on protein composition (Tellez *et al.,* 2014).

Nutrigenomics clarify that the system of gene interacts with nutrients and how DNA and genetic code affect the needs for certain nutrients and quantities (German, 2005 and Miggiano *et al.,* 2006) and helps to understand the nutritional effect on gene expression. To explore the importance of diet and diet formulation it is a need to understand physiological, biochemical and metabolic pathways and gene expression in livestock including poultry (Banerjee *et al.,* 2015).

## Application of Nutrigenomics in Animal Sector

Application of genomic principles in a nutrigenomics helps to formulate a specific association between nutrients and genetic factors. Nutrigenomics could be applicable to determine a personal diet (individual nutritional requirements based on the genetic makeup of the person), clarifies diet related disease and could find out the associated genes that are concerned in diet- gene interaction, detects polymorphism of gene that may have significant nutritional and environmental factors on genetic expression. Also through the application of single nucleotide polymorphism clarifies the different responses to same nutrient by different individuals and explores the effect of genetic variation on the interaction between diet and disease.

Nutrigenomics will relate optimal diet to choose from many and different nutritional availability while nutrigenetics will formulate information for identifying the optimal diet for a given subject (Ordovas *et al.,* 2004). On the road to define the optimal diets for an individual's; it is a need to clarify the health status at molecular stage with the consideration of metabolic and epidemiological studies. Nutrigenomics correlates diet, health and genomics in term of phenotypic effect also include different omics such as proteomics and transcriptomics (Tellez *et al.,* 2014). Through different molecular and nutritional researches there are several factors including environmental which are associated with animal health.

To evaluate the interaction between diets and genes, DNA microarray techniques and quantitative real-time Polymerase Chain Reaction (PCR) and DNA sequencing can be applied (Morozova *et al.,* 2008). The interaction between diets and genes could be evaluated through DNA microarray techniques and quantitative real- time polymerase chain reaction (PCR). Now a days, microarray or DNA chip technology in nutrigenomics research enables to screening large numbers of genes and giving comprehensive picture of the variation of gene expression patterns.

Nutrigenomics in livestock agriculture can easily be employed with minimum cost and may be effective in increment of growth rate, milk production and composition, feed usage and carcass composition, disease resistance, enhanced reproductive and prolificacy enhancement. Generally, nutrigenomics can bridge the gap between genetic profile and feeding for better conversion efficiency in livestock production and productivity (Figure 9.1).

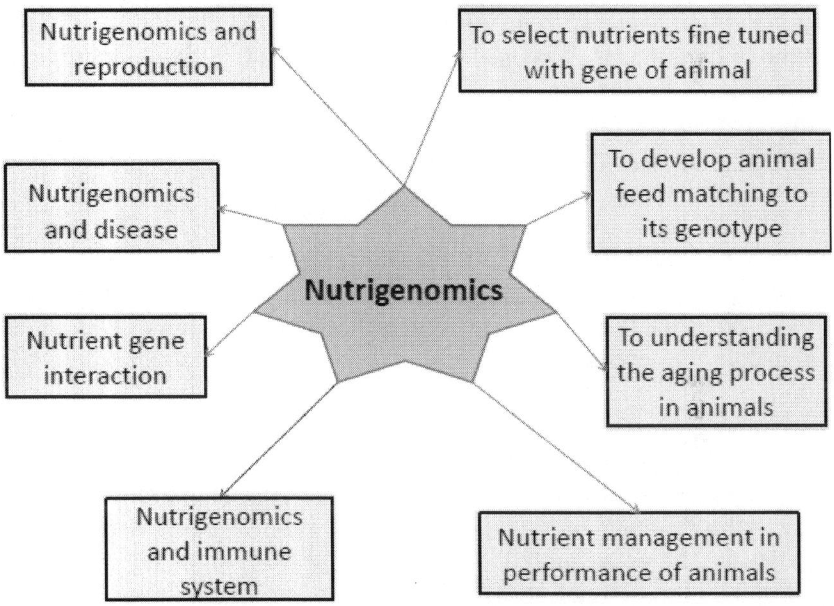


**Figure 9.1. Schematic Overview of Integration of Omics Technology in Animal Feeding and Nutritional Research.**

## Nutrigenomics in Poultry and Swine Industry

Nutrigenomics approach is carefully selecting nutrients for fine tuning genes and DNA presents in every cell and every tissue of an animal. It is possible to measure the effects of certain nutritional supplements and how they alter the gene interaction of the body using gene chips that contain the genetic code of animal. Demand of meat (poultry and pork) is increasing rapidly due to globalization and increasing population all over the world and due to increase of cereal cost there is a need to consider the nutrigenomics approach.

## Current Progress of the Area with Emphasis to Developing Countries

Area of research in farm animals were mainly focusing on nutrient requirement of animal for maintenance, production and reproduction, diet formulation in order to optimize feed and production efficiency. Efficient nutrient utilization has strong correlation with farm animal production and which it relates with methane production, proper utilization of nutrient and competition in use for feed, food or fuel (Jansman *et al.,* 2015). Hence, the intricate interactions between diet and many aspects of animal health are poorly understood.

There is a considerable interest in the application of molecular genetics technology for the inheritable traits of growth rate, body weight, carcass merit, feed intake, milk yield and composition (Spelman *et al.,* 1998). Proteomics and metabolite techniques can be used for determination of protein and metabolite composition of livestock products. Omics techniques like transcriptomics, proteomics and metabolomics helps the current animal production to highlight the metabolic, nutrient status of an animal and act to adjust the metabolism to the nutrient status (Jansman *et al.,* 2015). Feed cost comprises the variable expense in animal production system making feed efficiency an important economic consideration (Bernabucci *et al.,* 2004). The gene expression of etiology of fatty liver in dairy cows at calving and gene expression of gluconeogenesis in early lactation in cows (Greenfield *et al.,* 2000), transcriptome analysis of cattle muscle identifies potential markers for skeletal muscle growth rate and major cell types were understood (Guo *et al.,* 2015).

## Challenges and Opportunities

The demand for animal products has been increasing in line with urbanization and population growth. In addition, some of the cereal feeds used for animal production could also be served for humans as well. This phenomena needs an innovation solution to convert small amount of feed for a production, this may be possible via omics' technology. Optimization of productivity and efficiency in nutrition utilization could be possible. However, there is limitation in nutrigenomic information how to effectively analyze and correlate genes and nutrition conversion in livestock production. To manipulate this, the genetic potential is partially utilized, the utilization of most nutrients appears to be low and hence, there is a huge variation in performance. From a Nitrogenomics point of view, it is possible to expect to change the way we feed and manage livestock and poultry (Dawson *et al.,* 2006).

Environmental, cultural and economic factors also play an essential role in individual food choices and accessibility (Fenech *et al.,* 2011). Malnutrition in the form of under nutrition or obesity can also modify gene expression and genome stability, resulting in changes in phenotype, and hence it is difficult to choose one population as a reference. The availability of genomic information is important to determine a specific nutrient under specific condition. Usage of this genomic information raises questions on how to apply such knowledge and how to use such information. Interpretation and consideration of genotype of individual for nutritional suggestion financial, ethical and customer preference aspect may affect the revolution of nutrition (Lynnette *et al.,* 2016).

## Conclusion

Nutrient and food components can affect gene expression/regulation directly and indirectly, transcription and plays a regulatory role in intermediate metabolites of signaling pathways, with positive or negative effects. Now a days, microarray or DNA chip technology in nutrigenomics research enables to screening large numbers of genes and giving comprehensive picture of the variation of gene expression patterns which allowed researchers for examination of nutrient effects which were not possible in the past. There is a considerable interest in the application of molecular genetics technology for the inheritable traits of growth rate, body weight, carcass merit, feed intake, milk yield and composition. Nutrigenomics can only provide part of the solution in response to non genetic factors involved in an individual's health and production.

## REFERENCES

Andersen, H.J., Oksbjerg, N.Y., and Therkildsen, M. (2005). Feeding and meat quality-A future approach. *Meat Science,* **70**(3): 543-554.

Banerjee, G., Pal, R., and Ray, A.K. (2015). Applications of Nutrigenomics in Animal Sectors: A Review. *Asian J Anim Vet Adv,* **10**: 489-499.

Benítez, R., Núñez, Y., Óvilo, C. (2017). Nutrigenomics in Farm Animals. J Investig Genomics 4(1): 00059. DOI: 10.15406/jig.2017.04.00059.

Bernabucci, U., Ronchi, B., Basirico, L., Pirazzi, D. and Rueca, F. (2004). Abundance of mRNA of apolipoprotein B100, apolipoprotein E and microsomal triglyceride transfer protein in liver from periparturient cows. *J Dairy Sci,* **87**: 2881-2888.

Dawson, K.A. (2006). Nutrigenomics: Feeding the genes for improved fertility. *Anim Reprod Sci.,* **96**: 312-322.

Fenech, M., El-Sohemy, A., Cahill, L., Ferguson, L.R. and French, T.A. (2011). Nutrigenetics and Nutrigenomics: Viewpoints on the Current Status and Applications in Nutrition Research and Practice. *J Nutrigenet Nutrigenomics,* 69-89.

German, J.B. (2005). Genetic dietetics: nutrigenomics and the future of dietetics practice. *J Am Diet Assoc,*: 530-531.

Greenfield, R.B., Cevana, M.J. and Donkin, S.S. (2000). Changes in *m*RNA expression for gluconeogenic enzymes in liver of dairy cattle during the transition to lactation. *J Dairy Sci,* **83**: 1228-1236.

Jansman, A.J.M. and Pas, M.F.W. (2015). Techniques for evaluating nutrient status in farm animals. Wageningen U.R. (University and Research Centre) Livestock Research, *Livestock Research Report,* 846.

Jiang, Z.Y., Zhong, W.J., Zheng, C.T., Lin, Y.C., Yang, L., *et al.* (2010) Conjugated linoleic acid differentially regulates fat deposition in backfat and longissimus muscle of finishing pigs. J Anim Sci 88 (5): 1694-1705.

Li, W.J., Zhao, G.P., Chen, J.L., Zheng, M.Q. and Wen, J. (2009). Influence of dietary vitamin E supplementation on meat quality traits and gene expression related to lipid metabolism in the beijing-you chicken. *Br Poult Sci,* **50**: 188-198.

Lynnette, R.F., De, C.R., Görman, U., Allayee, H. and Kohlmeier, M. (2016). Guide and Position of the International Society of Nutrigenetics/Nutrigenomics on Personalised Nutrition: Part 1-Fields of Precision Nutrition. *J Nutrigenet Nutrigenomics,* **9**: 12-27.

Miggiano, G.A. and De, S. (2006).Nutritional genomics: toward a personalized diet US National Library of Medicine, National institutes of health. *La clin Ter,* **157**: 355-361.

Morozova, O. and Marra, M.A. (2008). Applications of next-generation sequencing technologies in functional genomics. *Genomics,* **92**: 255-264.

Ordovas, J.M. and Mooser, V. (2004). Nutrigenomics and nutrigenetics. *Curr Opin Lipidol,* **15**: 101-108.

Schmidt, C.W. (2007) Biodiesel: Cultivating alternative fuels. *Environ Health Perspect,* **115**: A87-A91.

Spelman, R.J. and Bovenhuis, H. (1998). Moving from QTL experimental results to the utilization of QTL in breeding programmes. *Anim Genet,* **29**: 77-84.

Swanson, K.S., Schook, L.B. and Fahey, G.C. (2003). Nutritional genomics: Implications for companion animals. *J Nutr,* **133**: 3033-3040.

Tellez, G., Latorre, J.D., Kuttappan, V.A., Kogut, M.H. and Wolfenden, A. (2014). Utilization of rye as energy source affects bacterial translocation, intestinal viscosity, microbiota composition and bone mineralization in broiler chickens. *Front Genet,* **5**: 339.

Wang, J., Chen, L., Li, P., Li, X. and Zhou, H. (2008). Gene expression is altered in piglet small intestine by weaning and dietary glutamine supplementation. *J. Nutr,* **138**: 1025- 1032.

## Chapter 10

# Nutritional Management to Avoid Common Metabolic Disorders in Livestock

*Amita Tiwari and Devendra Kumar Gupta*

*Department of Veterinary Medicine,*
*College of Veterinary Science and Animal Husbandry,*
*Nanaji Deshmukh Veterinary Science University, Jabalpur, Madhya Pradesh*

Among domestic animals, the metabolic diseases achieve their greatest importance in dairy animals. These are diseases of livestock caused by productivity practices when the body reserves on calcium, magnesium or energy can not meet the metabolic needs. They are very important in places where high producing animals are required, *e.g.* in diary industry. In cattle, metabolic diseases include ketosis, milk fever (parturient paresis), fat cow syndrome (fatty liver syndrome) and hypomagnesaemia. All these can produce an acute, temporary, but potentially fatal deficiency. The high producing dairy animals always verges on abnormal homeostasis and the breeding and feeding of dairy animals for high milk yield is etiologically related to metabolic diseases so common in these animals. In dairy animals, the incidence of metabolic diseases is highest in the period commencing at calving and extending until the peak of lactation (periparturient period) is reached. Most of metabolic diseases result from nutritional deficiencies during the crucial period from late pregnancy to peak lactation when body reserves can not cope up the metabolic demands.

## Lipid-Related Metabolic Disorders in Periparturient Dairy Cows

Plasma NEFA concentrations increase prior to and at parturition, resulting in increased fatty acid uptake by the liver, fatty acid esterification, and triglyceride storage. Liver triglyceride concentration increases four- to fivefold between d 17 prior to calving and d 1 following calving. Increases in liver triglyceride following calving do not appear to be dramatic. Severity of fatty liver 1 d postpartum is correlated negatively with feed intake 1 d pre partum. Export of newly synthesized triglyceride as very low density lipoprotein occurs slowly in ruminants and is a major factor in the development of fatty liver. Nutritional strategies to minimize the elevation in plasma NEFA prior to calving results in lower liver triglyceride at calving. Fatty liver probably precedes clinical spontaneous ketosis. Liver triglyceride to glycogen ratio may be used to predict susceptibility of cows to ketosis. Consequently, strategies to reduce liver triglyceride at calving may decrease incidence of ketosis. Research to determine methods to reduce fatty acid delivery to the liver or to enhance hepatic export of very low density lipoprotein near calving is warranted. Identification of the cause for the slow rate of assembly and secretion of hepatic very low density lipoprotein in ruminants will be required to assess the feasibility of increasing export of very low density lipoprotein.

## Energy Metabolism Associated Disease

### Fat Cow Syndrome

Excess energy (concentrates, corn silage, some hays) fed during the dry period may cause obese cows near calving time. These ¯too fat cows are more susceptible to a number of other metabolic problems (milk fever, ketosis, displaced abomasum, retained placenta, metritis) and the chance of dying is more likely.

It is not uncommon in some operations for overweight Holstein cows to weigh 1,600 to 2,000 pounds, which frequently creates problems. Feeding strategy is recommended to restore lost body condition during late lactation. Not only will this practice help avoid severely overweight cows, but feed conversion into body tissue is more efficient during late lactation, compared to the dry period. Try to achieve a body condition score of about 3.5 at dry-off, and then maintain this condition during the dry period to minimize the incidence of fat cow syndrome.

### Ketosis

This metabolic disease occurs most frequently in early lactation and may be associated with other problems, such as fat cow syndrome, retained placenta, mastitis, metritis, and displaced abomasum. Ketosis-positive cows always should be examined for these other complicating factors. Ketosis signs include off-feed, weight loss, decreased milk production, listlessness and other unusual signs. Ketosis is best prevented by keeping cows in good condition, *but not fat*, during the dry period. Begin to ¯lead feed grain 10-15 days prior to calving. Increase the grain ration about 1 pound per day up to a maximum level of 15 pounds. Feed changes during the first six weeks of lactation also should be gradual. During lactation, good quality, high energy, palatable feeds should be fed.

## Calcium/Phosphorus Metabolism Diseases/Complications

### Hypocalcemia (Milk Fever)

It generally occurs at or near calving. It is caused by a large calcium demand at the onset of milk production. The cow is unable to meet this calcium demand, due to ration imbalance, Vitamin D influence or parathyroid gland activity, all of which influence regulation of these metabolites during the dry period. Milk fever signs include staggering, inability to rise, muscular weakness, recumbency (laying down) and a subnormal temperature. The following are other problems that may occur due to milk fever:

1. Difficult calving due to muscular weakness that prevents proper labor.
2. Increased chance of uterine prolapse.
3. Tendencies to increase retained placentas.
4. Increased possibility of metritis (uterine infection).
5. Decreased reproductive performance.
6. Increased tendencies to bloat due to rumen muscle tone loss (atony).
7. Greater numbers of abomasal displacements.
8. Much greater risk of ketosis.
9. Considerably greater risk of developing mastitis.
10. Greater risk of other infectious disease.
11. Decreased milk production.
12. Reduced total productive life in the herd.

The after-effects of hypocalcemia conditions are very costly, illustrating the importance of prevention.

## Disease Control of Calcium/Phosphorus Imbalance

The most important and critical time to adjust imbalances causing metabolic problems due to calcium/phosphorus is the month prior to calving.

Requirements include:

- ✰ Limit pre-calving calcium intake. Feeding an excess tends to inhibit normal calcium mobilization from the bones.
- ✰ Total calcium requirement for a 1,200-pound dry cow is approximately 40 gm/day. In general, try not to feed in excess of 0.40 per cent calcium (percent of ration dry matter) to dry cows.
- ✰ Nutrients fed to the cow should be generally low in calcium. For example, alfalfa contains approximately 6 grams of calcium per pound. The calcium intake could easily be in excess if alfalfa was the only feed.

- ☆ If milk fever problems persist, limit total calcium to less than 60 grams per head per day. If herd problems of hypocalcemia continues on, reduce the precalving ration further to 20-25 gm per day.
- ☆ Avoid feeding high phosphorus levels. Phosphorus requirement is 28-30 gm/day and should be maintained near this level. Try to feed approximately 0.24 per cent phosphorus as a percentage of ration dry matter.
- ☆ Keep pre-calving potassium levels as low as possible because high forage potassium levels may predispose cows to milk fever regardless of calcium intake. Forages low in potassium are usually low in calcium. If this is not practical, consult with a nutritionist about feeding anionic salts to dry cows.

## Diet

Healthy, well fed animals may tolerate many external risk factors but does chronically underfeed is not able to compensate. The major disorders affecting the fresh cow are usually the result of nutrition and feed management problems. Nutritional imbalances, deficiencies, or erratic management of feeding programs for dairy cows can create large numbers and various types of health problems generally categorized as metabolic diseases.

Dry matter intake typically declines; in the final week before parturition, restricted water intake or poor quality water, rapid feed changes, transportation, poor quality forage that is too woody, preventive measures such as vaccination (performed in late gestation), particularly if they are held off feed for the procedure. This declines in dry matter intake and changes in endocrine profiles contribute to elevated blood nonesterified fatty acids which have been related to the occurrence of lipid related metabolic diseases such as fatty liver and ketosis.

High calcium intake during dry period (over 100-125 g/cow/day) tends to increase the problem as high calcium depresses the activity of paratharmones and its gland and make animal more prone for parturient paresis. Hence low calcium (8 g/day/450 kg B. Wt.) and high phosphorus diet is recommended during dry period.

Acidic pH in gut is required for calcium absorption. If cations (sodium and potassium) are more in diet, it increases the risk of milk fever although high proportion of anions (chloride and sulphur) in diet decreases the risk.

Hypomagnesaemia in cattle and sheep is common when feeding of most winter season grasses, young cereal crops and corn stover. Nitrogen fertilizer increases ammonia concentration which impairs magnesium absorption and makes them susceptible to hypomagnesaemic tetany. Optimal sodium potassium ratio (Na:K :: 5:1) in rumen is required to transport magnesium across the epithelium of fore stomach by an active Na linked ATPase dependent transport system. If this ratio disturb, increases the chances of hypomagnesemic tetany. Calves kept on whole milk diet are on risk of hypomagnesemic tetany as milk is poor source of magnesium.

Ingestion of large quantity of rape, turnip and other cruciferous plants (low in phosphorus) increases risk for postparturient haemoglobinuria. Phosphorus deficient soil is common predisposing cause of post parturient haemoglobinuria

Fatty liver syndrome is common when system of challenge feeding of dairy cows is practiced with high energy ration.

## Body Condition Score

Cow body condition evaluation is important because reproductive efficiency is considerably reduced in extremely thin or too-fat cows'. The too-fat cows have more problems at post-calving (retained placentas, metritis, cystic ovaries) while too-thin cows usually have breeding problems due to prolonged time lapse before resuming normal heat cycles (30-40 days post-calving). Body condition scores (1 as too thin and 5 at too fat) for lactating cows, at peak production, should not drop below 2.5 and should be dried off at 3.5 and maintain this score throughout the dry period. The body condition score of the animal entering into late gestation is important.

- Animals that are very thin have little fat or muscle reserves to draw upon and are then at increased risk despite a good ration.
- Very fat animals will readily use body fat reserves in late gestation but also experience decreased voluntary intakes, thus predisposing them to formation of ketone bodies in ketosis that further suppress appetite.
- High body condition score increases risk for parturient paresis, udder edema and ketosis.

Chapter 11

# Nutritional Strategies to Alleviate Heat Stress in Dairy Animals

*Anand Jain, Aditya Mishra and Jyotsana Shakkarpude*

*Department of Veterinary Physiology and Biochemistry, College of Veterinary Science and Animal Husbandry, Nanaji Deshmukh Veterinary Science University, Jabalpur, Madhya Pradesh*

## Introduction

India ranks first in the world milk production with annual milk production of 132.4 million and contribute about 16 per cent to the world milk production (BAHS, 2014). Dairying has been playing a major role for the rural people by providing livelihoods. However, environmental extremes are the major constraints in dairy animals which severely affect milk production. Because of the climate change effects, summer temperatures have been increasing worldwide and this trend will continue in near future also. Among the livestock animals dairy animals are likely to be impacted greatly by the effects of climate change. The international panel for climate changes (IPCC, 2007) predicts that by 2100 the increase in global average surface temperature may be between 1.8°C to 4.0°C. India is also experiencing increased average temperatures and humidity and more hot spells recently. Severe heat stress in dairy animals is observed due to hot days, followed by hot nights as cows accumulate heat and cannot adequately dissipate this body heat. In extremes deaths from heat exhaustion may occur during very hot and humid periods. As the animal productivity decreases during the summer due to consequences of heat stress, it is one of the costliest issues facing animal producers and certainly one of the primary constraints to efficient and profitable animal husbandry in developing countries. The thermoneutral zone (TNZ) of dairy animals ranges from 16°C to 25°C, within which they maintained a physiological body temperature of 38.4-39.1°C. However, air temperatures above 25-37°C in a tropical climate like in India, it enhance heat gain beyond that lost from the body and induces heat stress. Heat stress is the state at which physiological mechanisms get activated to maintain an animal's body thermal balance, when it is exposed to intolerable temperature and humidity. The environmental factors associated with heat stress which affect the physiological systems regulating thermal balance are primarily ambient temperature, relative humidity and radiant energy. HS results in increases body surface temperature, respiration rate, heart rate and rectal temperature which in turn affects feed intake, production and reproductive efficiency of animals. However, the animal being homeotherms can resist to HS up to some extents depending on species, breed and productivity. Among dairy animals, goats were the most adapted species to imposed HS in terms of production, reproduction and also to disease resistance. The sensitivity of dairy cattle to HS increases with increase in milk production which might be due increases in metabolic heat output with increase production levels in dairy animals.

Three management strategies have been identified to minimize the effects of HS are physical modification of the environment, genetic development of heat tolerant breeds and improved feeding and nutritional management practices. The nutritional strategies should be aimed at maintaining water balance, nutrients and electrolytes intake and to satisfy the special needs during heat stress such as vitamins and minerals.

## Effects of Heat Stress on Dairy Animals

The most common signs of heat stress in cows are:

- Reduced feed intake
- Reduced milk yield and milk fat
- Reduced activity
- Increased respiration rate
- Increased body temperature
- Impaired reproductive performance.

### Dry Matter Intake

In heat stress dry matter intake is reduced by 9 – 13 per cent. The reduced feed intake is mainly due to panting, which reduces cud chewing, slows the breakdown of feed, and reduces the amount of water and buffers from saliva reaching the rumen. Early lactating and higher yielding cows are affected more quickly and severely. In grazing animals, standing in the shade to keep cool also restricts grazing time and decreases intake.

### Milk Production

As the feed intake decreases, so does the milk production. Milk production drops further if water is limiting. Cows divert water from milk production to facilitate cooling.

### Milk Fat

Milk fat content declines by up to 0.3 per cent units during summer.

### Fertility/Reproduction

During the summer season fertility rate is decreased in dairy animals as compared to winter season. Early embryonic deaths account for significant losses in heat stressed cows.

### Rumen Health

Recent research indicates that heat stressed cows have reduced rate of passage, lower rumen pH, higher rumen ammonia and change in volatile fatty acids. This affect appears to be independent of changes in dry matter intake. Heat stress can slow rumen contractions, which in turn slows digestion.

## Nutritional Strategies to Alleviate Heat Stress

There are several nutritional strategies which can be used to mitigate heat stress in dairy animals.

### 1. Water

It is most important nutrient for dairy cows subjected to heat stress. Milk contains about 87 per cent water and it is critical for dissipation of excess body heat. Moreover, water intake is highly correlated with milk yield and dry matter intake. Increasing water availability to cows is one of most important strategy to alleviate heat stress.

The consumption of water increases sharply as the environmental temperature increases because of greater water losses from sweating and from water vaporization with more rapid respiratory rates (panting), both efforts aimed at increasing evaporative cooling for the cow. So, the normal water supply recommendations are inadequate in the summer. Water intake increases by up to 50 per cent as the THI approaches 80. Supply unlimited clean, cool and fresh water under shade within easy walking distance for the cow. So, place extra water points close to where the cows spend most of the time. Increase the number of drinking places. Provide water of low temperature (< 15°C) and clean troughs every 2 days.

As feed intake is markedly decreased during heat stress, a common strategy is to increase the energy and nutrient densities (increased concentrates and supplemental fat) of the diet. In addition to the energy balance, reducing the fiber content of the diet is thought to improve the cow's thermal balance and may reduce body temperature. However, increasing ration concentrates should be considered with care as heat stressed cows are highly prone to rumen acidosis. The nutritional needs of the cow change during heat stress, and ration reformulation to account for decreased DMI, the need to increase nutrient density, changing nutrient requirements, avoiding nutrient excesses and maintenance of normal rumen function is necessary.

## 2. Supplementation of Fat

Increasing the amount of dietary fat has been a widely accepted strategy in order to reduce basal metabolic heat production. The heat increment of fat is less (up to 50 per cent) than the forages, so it is seemingly a rational decision to supplement additional fat and reduce fiber content of the diet.

## 3. Feeding of Fiber

One common nutritional strategy involves reducing dietary fiber during an increased heat-load. However, adequate fiber in the diet is essential to maintain rumen health, and high quality forage helps to maintain feed intake. NRC (2001) recommended that minimum dietary neutral detergent fiber (NDF) of 25 per cent with the proportion of NDF from roughages equaling 75 per cent of total NDF. However, its digestion and metabolism create more heat than compared to concentrates. Lower fibre, high grain diets may reduce metabolic heat production and contribute to lower heat load in the animal.

## 4. Protein Intake

Heat stress reduces feed intake, it is necessary to increase the protein level of the ration. However, the proportion of the dietary protein that must be provided as rumen un-degradable protein (bypass protein) must be increased, since the net passage of microbial protein from the rumen declines with lower DM intake. The oversupply of rumen degradable protein will lead to its inefficient use in the rumen which in turn will require the animal to expend energy to convert this wasted protein (as nitrogen) to urea which will largely be excreted in the urine.

## 5. Organic Trace Mineral Supplementation

Minerals such as zinc (Zn), chromium (Cr) and selenium (Se) have been recommended as external antioxidants in the management of oxidative stress cause by heat stress. Conventionally, inorganic minerals are used in diet, because they are cost- effective and readily available, but are relatively inferior to organic minerals due to poor bioavailability. In the gastro-intestinal tract, the inorganic minerals chelate with phytic acid complex and reduce their rate of absorption and consequently affect the tissue uptake of minerals. In contrast, organic minerals are devoid of free divalent cations for chelation in the intestinal lumen with phytic acid and hence they are differently metabolized facilitating enhanced absorption. It is in this context that organic minerals could be advantageously incorporated in diet at lower level than the inorganic sources for realizing higher mineral bio availability and lower excretion to address the environmental concerns due to less addition of inorganic forms and better absorption. A single or blend of organic trace mineral (OTM) in diets has been shown to have multiple beneficial effects.

Supplementation of zinc (Zn) in diet is of particular interest because they function predominantly as catalyst in many enzyme and hormone system that are associated with growth, immune response and have antioxidant activity.

### Selenium Supplementation

Selenium (Se) plays an important role in immune function, production of immunoglobulin and as a part of antioxidant system. Natural and synthetic antioxidants in the feed as well as optimal levels of minerals, principally selenium, help to maintain efficient levels of endogenous antioxidants in tissues. Selenium protects tissues against oxidative stress, as it is a component of the glutathione peroxidase (GPX) enzyme, which destroys free radicals in the cytoplasm.

### Chromium Supplementation

Chromium (Cr) is an essential element required for carbohydrate, fat and protein metabolism. Immunological function has been enhanced by trivalent Cr and its effects seem more pronounced during times of stress. Dietary chromium supplementation increases the growth rate, feed efficiency and improves milk yield as well as milk quality. Chromium is a micronutrient that facilitates insulin action on glucose, lipid, and protein metabolism. Spears *et al.* (2012) reported that heifers supplemented with increasing amounts of chromium had increased insulin sensitivity, suggesting that chromium plays an essential role in glucose metabolism in ruminants.

Because glucose use predominates during heat stress, chromium supplementation may improve thermal tolerance or production in heat-stressed animals. In addition, supplementing heat-stressed early lactation dairy cows with chromium reduced the degree of weight loss, improved milk production, reduced plasma NEFA concentrations and improved rebreeding rates (Mirzaei *et al.*, 2011). Dietary inorganic chromium supplementation in summer-exposed buffalo calves improved heat tolerance, immune status and potency of insulin hormone (Kumar *et al.*, 2015).

## 6. Vitamins Supplementation

Vitamins such as A, E (as a antioxidant) and niacin supplementation are used to reduce the heat stress in dairy animals. In order to reduce the negative effects of environmental stress, vitamins A, C and E are generally used in hot diets', because of their anti-stress effects and also because their concentrations are lower during HS. Dietary supplementation of vitamin A reduces the detrimental effect of HS. The supplementation is also favourable for the immunity of heat-stressed animals, and could alleviate the oxidative injuries induced by heat exposure and immune challenge. Vitamin A, together to vitamin E and trace elements (in particular Se, Cu and Zn) are among the micronutrients playing important roles on mammary gland immunity and health, in particular during stress conditions.The supplementation with trace elements and vitamins above National Research Council recommendation had positive effects on reproductive and lactation performance of high producing dairy cows kept under HS condition. In heat-stressed animals supplemented with ascorbic acid, a reduction of the respiratory quotient by emphasising a rise in fatty acid oxidation over the increase in protein-derived gluconeogenesis. Selenium and vitamin E supplemented parenteral in dairy cows during hot weather can alleviate the effects of HS, particularly for night- time feeding. Among vitamins, niacin was studied for its action on the vasodilatation in the mammalian and for its role in lipid metabolism. Niacin is a subcutaneous vasodilator in a many species and was studied in order to obtain a reduction of body temperature. However, niacin is rapidly metabolised in the rumen resulting in poor delivery to the small intestine. Niacin helps to alleviate HS both by increasing evaporative heat loss from the body and also by reducing the effects of heat at the cell level. Feeding protected niacin increased free plasma niacin levels, evaporative heat loss during peak thermal load and associated with a small but detectable reduction in rectal and vaginal temperatures in dairy cows experiencing a mild thermal load with variable effect on milk production (Zimbelman *et al.,* 2013).

## 7. Dietary Cation Anion Difference (DCAD)

Dietary cation anion difference (DCAD) is the difference between certain dietary minerals nominated as cations (Na, K) and anions (Cl, S) on the basis of charges they carry and is usually measured as milliequivalents of (Na+K)-(Cl+S) per kilogram of DM (Sarwar *et al.,* 2007). Wildman *et al.* (2007) stated that keeping the DCAD at a healthy lactating level (200 to 300 mEq/kg DM) remains a good strategy during the warm summer months. Animal productivity is influenced more by the difference between these cations and anions than their individual effects when fed as a sole independent mineral source. In addition, Shahzad *et al.* (2008) reported that a diet having DCAD 330 mEq/kg DM has promoted feed consumption, water intake and resulted in greater milk yield and milk fat in early lactating buffaloes.

## 8. Supplementation of Electrolyte

Bovines utilize potassium as their primary osmotic regulator of water secretion from sweat glands. As a consequence, potassium requirements are increased (1.4 to 1.6 per cent of DM) during the summer, and this should be adjusted for in the diet. Supplementation of electrolyte relieved oxidative stress and improved cell mediated immunity in heat stressed buffaloes. In addition, dietary levels of sodium and magnesium should be increased as they compete with potassium for intestinal absorption.

## 9. Supplementation of Rumen Fermentation Modifiers

Monensin is a well-described rumen fermentation modifier that increases the production of propionate, which is predominate gluconeogenic precursor in ruminants and thus improve the glucose status of heat-stressed cows. The use of live yeast cultures (Saccharomyces cerevisiae), has been extensively used to enhance nutrient utilization in ruminant animals (Francia *et al.,* 2008). The yeast culture supplementation increased feed intake and increased milk production during heat stress.

### 10. Barn Climate

Install and use appropriate fans Install and use showers, water spray producing devices, or sprinklers Increase the number of sprinkling and drying cycles per day

## Conclusion

Dairy animals are more sensitive to heat stress, which has significant economic impact for the farmers in terms of decreased productivity and health problems. Implementing heat stress mitigation strategies is crucial to minimize fiscal losses. In addition to physical environment management, nutritional strategies can be implemented to ameliorate heat stress induced losses.

Nutritional strategies to alleviate heat stress in dairy animals are summarized below:

- ☆ Water is the most important nutrient of all to minimize heat stress, provide access to plenty of clean fresh water. Ensure an adequate source of cool, fresh water. As temperatures rise into the mid-90s, dairy cows will increase their water intake by as much as 50 percent.
- ☆ Encourage maximum DM intake and increase density of energy and other nutrients to compensate for reduced DM intake.
- ☆ Supplement fat to the diet to improve energy density and to improve efficiency.
- ☆ Use high quality forages to increase the energy content of the diet and to maintain adequate rumination, and decreases the heat of fermentation associated with feeding lower-quality forages. As protein quality is important during hot weather, increase rumen un-degradable protein in ration and avoiding excessive rumen degradable protein.
- ☆ Consider specific supplementations such as niacin, chromium, selenium, antioxidants, electrolytes and rumen fermentation modifiers that have proven beneficial during heat stress.
- ☆ Heat-stressed dairy cows should be fed adequate amounts of trace minerals and vitamins.
- ☆ Consider the addition of high-fat feeds, bypass fats or lower fiber feedstuffs.
- ☆ Alter feeding times to allow more feed intake at night, when it is cool.
- ☆ Consider adding a nutritional supplement to help support normal immune function

## REFERENCES


BAHS. 2014. Basic Animal Husbandry Statistics. Department of Animal Husbandry, Dairying and Fisheries, Ministry of Agriculture, Government of India, New Delhi.

Francia, A., Masucci, F., De Rosa, G., Varricchio, M.L. and Proto, V. (2008). Effects of Aspergillus oryzae extract and a Saccharomyces cerevisiae fermentation product on intake, body weight gain and digestibility in buffalo calves. *Animal Feed Science and Technology*, **140**: 67-77.

IPCC. 2007. The intergovernmental panel on climate change, 4th assessment report. Available from: http: //www.ipcc.ch/.

Kumar, M., Kaur, H., Deka, R.S., Mani, V., Tyagi, A.K. and Chandra, G. (2015). Dietary inorganic chromium in summer-exposed buffalo calves (Bubalus bubalis): effects on biomarkers of heat stress, immune status, and endocrine variables. *Biological Trace Element Research*, **167**: 18-27.

Mirzaei, M, Ghorbani, G.R., Khorvash, M., Rahmani, H.R. and Nikkhah, A. (2011). Chromium improves production and alters metabolism of early lactation cows in summer. *Journal of Animal Physiology and Animal Nutrition*, **95**: 81-89

NRC. 2001. Nutrient requirements of dairy cattle. 7th Revised Edition, National Research Council, National Academy Press, Washington, DC, USA.

Sarwar, M., Shahzad, M.A. and Nisa M. (2007). Nutrients intake, acid base status and growth performance of growing Thalli lambs fed varying level of dietary cation anion difference. *Asian Australasian Journal of Animal Science*. **20**: 1858-1864.

Shahzad, M.A., Sarwar, M. and Nisa, M. (2007). Nutrients intake, acid base status and growth performance of growing male buffalo calves fed varying level of dietary cation anion difference. *Livestock Science*. **111**: 136-143

Spears, J.W., Whisnant, C.S., Huntington, G.B. Lloyd, K.E., Fry, R.S., Krafka, K., Lamptey, A. and Hyda, J. (2012). Chromium propionate enhances insulin sensitivity in growing cattle. *Journal of Dairy Science*. **95**: 2037-2045.

Wildman, C.D., West, J.W. and Bernard, J.K. (2007). Effect of dietary cation-anion difference and dietary crude protein on performance of lactating dairy cows during hot weather. *Journal of Dairy Science*. **90**: 1842-1850

Zimbelman, R.B., Collier, R.J. and Bilby, T.R. (2013). Effects of utilizing rumen protected niacin on core body temperature as well as milk production and composition in lactating dairy cows during heat stress. *Animal Feed Science and Technology*. **180**: 26-33.

## Chapter 12

# Nutritional Approaches to Manipulate Ruminal Efficiency

*Anju Nayak, Joycee Jogi, Sanjay Shukla, Poonam Shakya and Smita Bordoloi*

*Department of Veterinary Microbiology, College of Veterinary Science and Animal Husbandry, Nanaji Deshmukh Veterinary Science University, Jabalpur, Madhya Pradesh*

Rumen is a black hole in which what is happening is not known. About 11 per cent of the world's livestock population lives in India. Contribution of livestock sector to the national economy in terms of Gross Domestic Product (GDP) is 4.1 per cent. Small ruminants contribute 10 per cent of total livestock sector contribution in GDP of India. Small ruminants are the source of livelihood for poor farmers. The low productivity of ruminants due to inadequate feed, water and poor health care are the main issues. In India ruminants are mostly fed roughage based diets mostly lignocellulosic crop residues like straw and stovers. They are only partially utilized by animals therefore there is a need to improve utilization of nutrients from poor quality feeds by nutritional, microbiological or biotechnological interventions. These efforts will definitely show the way to farmer in doubling their income.

None of the animal origin enzyme can degrade roughage based diets so these animals are dependent on microorganism present in rumen for degradation of lignocellulosic feeds. In other words we can say rumen is an anaerobic fermentation sac in which pre gastric microbial fermentation of lignocellulosic feeds take place. Cattle and other ruminants can degrade fibrous feedstus owing to the consortium of bacteria, protozoa, fungi and methanogens inhabiting their rumen and hindgut. This consortium ferments fiber and other feed components to short-chain fatty acids (SCFA) and in the process, generates ATP that fuels microbial growth (synthesis of cellular protein in particular). This microbial protein supplies 60 to 85 per cent of amino acids (AA) reaching the animals small intestine. Maximizing eciency of its production would consequently improve cattle productivity. Production of microbial protein is inecient because microbes do not direct all ATP toward growth. Rather, microbes can direct some ATP toward maintenance functions, synthesis of reserve carbohydrate or energy spilling (futile cycles that dissipate heat).

## Importance of Rumen Microbes

The rumen microbes biomass consists of bacteria (40-50 per cent), protozoa (40-50 per cent) and fungi (40-50 per cent). They act synergistically to degrade feed in the rumen. Archaea and bacteriophage helps indirectly in fermentation of feed. Bacteria, protozoa and fungi do not compete with each other on active sites of feed as they have distinctly different mode of action on fibrous feed. Protozoa engulf small fibrous feed particles by phagocytosis. The protozoa do not have intimate contact with the substrate, but they contribute significant portion of hydrolytic enzyme in rumen contents. The cellulolytic bacteria attach with the feed particle with the help of glycoprotein coat and excrete fibre degrading enzymes and create cavities on the surface of feed particles. The rumen fungi penetrate into the substrate and cut feed particles into several pieces, thereby increasing total surface area of feed on which either bacteria can act and hydrolyse or protozoa can engulf and hydrolyse the lignocellulosic feed into monosaccharides. The Archaea (methanogens) are responsible for conversion of carbon di oxide to methane by utilizing hydrogen generated during fermentation. This might be the reason that there is no hydrogen accumulation in the rumen gaseous phase inspite of the fact that a lot of hydrogen (600-800 litres in rumen of adult cow)is generated every day. Bacteriophages are responsible for high bacterial turnover in the rumen and make bacterial protein available to the host by lysing bacteria. Increasing the production of microbes in the rumen is the key to lifting milk production and composition. The microbes break down feed to produce volatile fatty acids, which are used by the cow as energy for maintenance and milk production. The rumen microbes are also digested and absorbed in the small intestine of the dairy cow as the main protein source for milk production, providing up to 70-90 per cent of a cow´s protein requirements.

## Importance of a Consistent Diet

Microbe populations take time to recover and build up after sudden feed changes. Forage fibre-digesting microbes may take 4-6 weeks to build up. Starch-digesting (grain-digesting) microbes take 4-5 days to build up. Lactic acid-producing bacteria (from slug feeding) take 2-4 hours to build up. If a cow's diet keeps changing every few days, the required microbes will not be present in sufficient numbers for optimum digestion. Therefore, a cow's diet should be as consistent as possible.

## Feed Additives

Initially feed additives were used to reduce the cost of the feed but now a day they are used to improve livestock production and health. The feed additives are broadly divided in following groups:

1. Probiotics
2. Prebiotics
3. Ionophores
4. Buffers
5. Enzymes
6. Plant secondary metabolites

### 1. Probiotics

Probiotics are "live microbial feed supplement which beneficially affects the host animal by improving its intestinal microbial balance". They are also classified as Direct Fed Microbes (DFM).The microbes which can be used as probiotics are beneficial bacteria like *Lactobacillus, Bacteroides, Bacillus, Pediococcus, propionibacterium, Streptococcus* and *Bifidobacterium* spp. *etc.*Most commonly used fungal cultures as probiotics are *Saccharomyces cervisiae* and *Aspergillus oryzae.* They modify rumen ecosystem by stimulating desirable microbes or inhibiting undesirable or harmful microbes. Modulating enzyme activity by increasing or decreasing different enzyme activities and create desired enzyme profile. Modulating immune system by increasing antibody production and macrophage activity.

### 2. Prebiotics

Prebiotics are nondigestible food ingredients that beneficially affect the host by selectively stimulating the growth and or activity of one or a limited number of bacteria in the colon thus improving host health. Commonly used prebiotics are oligosaccharides *i.e.*, fructo oligosaccharides (FOS), mannon oligosaccharides (MOS), lactulose and inulin. It is also widely used in animals to improve growth rate, increase milk yield, meat and egg production. Prebiotic consumption generally promotes *Lactobacillus* sp and *Bifidobacterium* sp growth in the intestine.

### 3. Ionophores

Ionophores are the organic compounds which is able to transport particular ions across a lipid membrane in a cell. They are the antimicrobial compounds which modify rumen ecosystem to benefit the animal by modulating Gram positive bacteria which are highly sensitive to ionophores. Most common ionophores are monensin, lasalocid, laidlomycin propionate, bambermycin and virginiamycin. Ionophores increases propionate production resulting in decrease acetate : propionate ratio. Decreases methane production, thus increases the energy utilization efficiency.

Decreases protein breakdown in rumen, reduces lactate accumulation. Reduces bloat, ketosis and improves the milk production efficiency.

## 4. Buffers

Buffers help to reduce the rumen acidity that commonly results from feeding diets designed for high milk production. They can increase dry matter intake, rumen microbial protein production, and fiber digestion, resulting in increased milk production and milkfat production. Sodium bicarbonate (bicarb) is the most common ruminal buffer.

## 5. Enzymes

Ruminants in spite of efficient fermentor are unable to extract all the nutrition from fibrous feed. To improve the fibre digestibility exogenous cell wall degrading enzymes are useful. The enzymes xylanases and cellulases are derived from fungi *viz. Trichoderma longibrachiatum, T. ressei, Aspergillus niger, A. oryzae* and bacteria belonging to *Bacillus* spp. All the benefits of improved feed digestibility can be achieved by enzymes.

## 6. Plant Secondary Metabolites

The secondary metabolites act as a defense mechanism for the plants due to their specific antimicrobial characterstics that is why they are explored as feed additives to modulate microbial ecosystem of gastrointestinal tract. The major secondary metabolites are tannins, saponins, alkaloids and essential oils. Plants rich in secondary metabolities shows anti methanogenic activity. Tannins can reduce the parasitic load of the animals, improves feed intake, nutrient utilization and ultimately growth of calves.

## Chapter 13

# Nutritional Approaches for Raising Product Quality in Ruminants

*Serlene Tomar and Simranjeet Kaur*

*Department of Livestock Products Technology,
College of Veterinary Science and Animal Husbandry,
Nanaji Deshmukh Veterinary Science University, Jabalpur, Madhya Pradesh*

Ruminant-derived foods are significant sources of medium-chain SFA and TFA, high-quality protein with most essential amino-acids, essential micronutrients and several bioactive lipids in the human diet. Milk and meat together provide about 60 and 55 per cent of the dietary intake of Ca and protein respectively. Meat makes a sizeable contribution to the intake of readily available Fe. However, public health policies recommend population-wide decrease in the consumption of fat, SFA and TFA, and higher intakes of PUFA. Moreover, in the recent years consumers have demanded healthier food and are paying more attention to the hedonistic aspect of food products. Milk and meat fatty acids composition and cholesterol content have important repercussions on human health. The animal dietary regimen strongly affects the FA composition of meat and meat colour, milk FA composition as well as its flavour. Therefore, altering the FA composition of ruminant-derived foods offers the opportunity to align the consumption of FA in human populations with public health policies without the need for substantial changes in eating habits.

## Milk and Meat Characteristics of Ruminants

Milk is a complex food, an almost indispensable part of the diets of infants and children. The quality of milk is determined mainly by the proportions of its individual components such as protein, fat, vitamins and carbohydrates. On an average, per cent fat composition of bovine milk is 4 per cent, out of which 97-98 per cent are triacylglycerides. The bovine milk FA typically contains a high percentage of SFA and MUFA comprising 69.4 per cent and 25 per cent, respectively. Further, 5 per cent PUFA is present in bovine milk which accounts for 2.3 per cent cis-PUFA and 2.7 per cent trans-PUFA. The most novel aspect reported to date concerning the composition of milk fat of ruminants concerns its content in CLA which range from 2.9 to 8.92 mg CLA/g of fat with many different isomers including predominantly cis-9, trans-11 CLA (75-90 per cent of total CLA). The TFA represent approximately 4 per cent of total milk FA.

Similarly, meat from ruminants is composed of water, fat, protein, minerals and a small proportion of carbohydrate. However, edible fats do not seem to be healthy, mostly due to their high content in SFA, low content of n-3 PUFA, and a variable content in TFA. The CLA content in fresh meat of ruminants range from 2.7-5.6 mg/g fat which makes up 79-92 per cent of c-9, t-11 isomer of CLA. All these features of ruminant edible fats are directly linked to the extensive biohydrogenation of the dietary unsaturated FA conducted by rumen microbiota.

## Dietary Fatty Acids and Chronic Disease

The relationship between dietary fat type, their intake and CVD has been extensively investigated, and strong and consistent associations have been reported. SFA generally raise total cholesterol and LDL cholesterol, individual FA in this family have markedly different effects. Myristic acid (14:0), palmitic acid (16:0) and lauric acid (12:0) have been associated with elevated plasma LDL-cholesterol concentrations in human subjects, while, stearic acid (18:0), has been shown to be essentially neutral. Palmitic acid, is quantitatively the most important SFA in milk and meat fat. Lauric acid and myristic acid in the human diet is derived from milk fat, thus consumption of dairy products is expected to have adverse effects on plasma cholesterol levels. Steffen and Jacobs (2003) studied the effect of a diet in human subjects over a period of 7 years and observed that consumers of low-fat milk have lower HDL-cholesterol levels and consumers of cream and butter have higher HDL-cholesterol levels. Further, substitution of SFA in metabolic studies revealed that both MUFA and PUFA lower plasma total cholesterol and LDL cholesterol with PUFA having a greater effect. However, high-PUFA diets have potentially-adverse health effects due to the formation of lipid peroxidation products. Epidemiological data and intervention studies in populations at risk of CHD indicate that EPA and DHA have substantial cardio- protective actions. High intakes of SFA may also be related to reduced insulin sensitivity, a key factor in the development of metabolic syndrome, higher risk of impaired glucose tolerance and higher fasting plasma glucose and insulin concentrations. A 3 month intervention study revealed that SFA rich diets (butter and margarine) impaired insulin sensitivity in human subjects while in MUFA diets (high- oleic sunflower oil) no such changes were observed indicating that SFA intakes need to be reduced and replacing them with MUFA and PUFA has potential benefits.

## Nutritional Approaches to Altering Milk Fat Composition

Milk fat typically contains (g/100 g) 70–75 SFA, 20–25 MUFA and 2–5 PUFA. FA secreted in milk originate from two sources, either by direct incorporation from the peripheral circulation or from *de novo* synthesis in the mammary gland using short- chain (2:0 and 4:0) precursors. Mammary *de novo* synthesis accounts for all 4:0–12:0, most of the 14:0 and typically about half the 16:0 secreted in milk, while all C18 and longer-chain FA are derived entirely from circulating plasma lipids. Bovine mammary gland has the ability to release FA from the synthetase complex at various stages, resulting in secretion of a wide range of short- and medium-chain FA. As a result of extensive biohydrogenation of dietary USFA by rumen bacteria, under most conditions 18:0 is the predominant long-chain FA available for absorption. However, increasing the supply of long-chain FA (chain length 18) to the mammary gland inhibits the synthesis of short- and medium-chain SFA. Unlike other ruminant tissues, the mammary gland cannot convert 16:0 to 18:0 by chain elongation. However, it is notable that secretion of oleic acid (cis-9-18: 1) in milk exceeds its uptake by the mammary gland as a result of the activity of stearoyl-CoA (D9) desaturase in mammary secretory cells that converts 18:0 to cis-9-18:1. Conversion of 18:0 to cis-9-18:1 is the predominant precursor-to-product process of the D9-desaturase, and about 40 per cent of the 18:0 taken up by the mammary gland is desaturated. As a result of the complex process by which milk FA originate, several nutritional approaches can be used to manipulate milk fatty acid composition. Both the amount and source of dietary lipid affect the extent and type of change that can be achieved.

### a) Supplementation of Dietary Oils/Oilseeds

Dietary plant oil or oilseed supplements are known to alter the FA composition of ruminant milk. The extent to which plant oils or oilseeds alter milk FA composition is dependent on several factors including the amount of oil in the diet, FA profile of the lipid supplement, form of lipid in the diet, processing of oilseeds and the composition of the basal diet. In general, these supplements increase milk fat 18:0, cis-9-18:1 and trans-18:1 contents due to extensive rumen metabolism of long-chain fatty acids, leading to an increased supply of biohydrogenation intermediates (both trans-18:1 and 18:2) and 18:0 to the mammary gland. Oils rich in oleic acid, linoleic acid and a- linolenic acid have been used to increase the concentrations of PUFA in milk.

Supplementing dairy cows with cracked whole rapeseed increases MUFA and reduces SFA. Dayani *et al.* (2004) observed an increase in linoleic acid and fat content in soyabean fed animals while 16:1 (trans-9), 16:1 (cis-9), 17:0, 17:1 (cis-9) FA were higher in sunflower seeds fed group. Soybean oil, flaxseed linseed, sunflower seeds, evening primrose oil (Hermansen *et al.*, 1995) supplementation reduce SFA and increase CLA concentration in milk fat. Fish oil has the potential to enhance the concentrations of long-chain n-3 PUFA, EPA and DHA in milk. Ruminal biohydrogenation of EPA and DHA is limited therefore, considerable amount of these

FA are available for incorporation in adipose tissue (Raes *et al.*, 2004). Fatahnia *et al.* (2008) observed an increase in total omega-3 FA in milk of Holstein cows fed diet containing 3 per cent fish oil.

### b) Pasture Grazing and Silage

Feeding system based on grazing is known to increase the proportion of beneficial FA. Milk from grazing ruminants contains lower proportions of SFA and higher trans-11 18:1, cis-9, trans-11 CLA, 18:2n-6 and 18:3n-3 concentrations. The extent of 18:2n-6 and 18:3n-3 enrichment in milk being related to grass maturity and lipid content. Compared with lowland pastures, milk from cows fed botanical diverse pastures typically contains lower 4:0 to 16:0 and higher 18:2n-6 and 18:3n-3 concentrations. Grazing or feeding of diversified grasses resulted in the production of milk fat richer in alpha lipoic acid and CLA. Increasing proportion of fresh grass in the diet induces a linear decrease in milk fat content and increase in USFA percentages at the expense of SFA. Replacing grass silage, grass hay or conserved lucerne with maize silage has variable effects on milk SFA content, but typically increases trans 18:1 and 18:2n-6 and lowers 18:3n-3 concentrations. Drying rather than ensiling has relatively minor effects on most FA, but consistently increases 18:3n-3 concentrations. Increasing the concentration of forage as compared to concentrate increased the concentration of total long chain fatty acids, UFA, MUFA and PUFA, while, SFA level reduced in the milk of crossbred cow. These authors concluded that cows producing 12-14 kg of milk/day could be best maintained on a dietary regimen of 70 per cent good quality roughage and 30 per cent concentrate to have the maximum production of human health beneficial conjugated linoleic acid.

### c) Supplementation of Bypass Fat/Rumen Protected Fat or Inert Fat

Role of the bypass fat in the rations of high producing dairy animals is very crucial for enhancing the energy density of ration. Supplementation of bypass fats in the diet of lactating cows generally decreases the proportions of short and medium chain SFA (C6:0 to C16:0) of milk fat due to reduction in *de novo* FA synthesis in mammary gland and increase in proportions of long chain FA (C18:1, C18:2, C18:3) due to increased uptake of preformed LCFA from blood. Similarly, an increase in the total USFA (32.01 to 39.22), LCFA (75.61 to 77.17), MUFA (29.68 to 33.53) and decrease in the total SFA (63.28 to 54.02) as percentage of the total fatty acids of milk has been reported in dairy cows supplemented with bypass fat in the diet. Renno *et al.* (2013) reported that supplementation of calcium salts of palm oil fatty acid reduced the proportion of caproic, caprylic and capric acids, while the concentration of palmitic, oleic, stearic, linoleic and linolenic acids in milk fat increased with increase in level of bypass fat supplementation in lactating crossbred cows.

## Nutritional Approaches to Altering Muscle Fatty Acid Composition

Generally, the fat in meats derived from ruminant animals is composed of (g/100 g) around 45–55 SFA, 45–50 MUFA and relatively minor amounts of PUFA. Much of the efforts in manipulating the FA composition in large ruminants and to a lesser extent in smaller ones has been directed towards increasing PUFA:SFA and enhancing n-3 PUFA:n-6 PUFA. Consistent with the nutritional strategies known to influence milk fat composition, the majority of studies in growing ruminants have examined the potential of forage species, forage conservation method and dietary plant oils, oilseeds, fish oil and marine algae supplements to alter muscle fatty acid composition. However, in contrast to milk, it is possible to influence the abundance of 20-carbon PUFA in tissue PL by supplementing the diet with sources of 18:2n-6 and 18:3n-3, as well as dietary supplements containing 20-carbon PUFA. The saturating effect of rumen can be overcome by feeding PUFA which are protected either chemically, by processing, or naturally *e.g.* within the seed coat. Some protection occurs when grain-based or grass-based diets are fed normally, leading to relatively more n–6 or n–3 fatty acids respectively. However, these produce different flavors in cooked meat due to the different oxidative changes occurring during storage and cooking. Rearing cattle or lambs on pasture rather than concentrate-based diets increases 18:3n-3 and the longer-chain derivatives in the PL fraction of muscle. Concentrates rich in 18:2n-6 result in higher concentrations of 18:2n-6 and associated longer-chain derivatives in the muscle of cattle and sheep. Both the amount of grass and duration of rearing on pasture influences the potential to enrich 18:3n-3, 20:5n-3 and 22:6n-3 in bovine muscle. Rearing on forage-based systems is associated with decrease in muscle 16:0 and total SFA and higher cis-9 18:1 concentrations as compared with n high-concentrate diets. Replacing grass silage with whole crop wheat silage or maize silage (increased the n-6:n-3 ratio of muscle.

A number of studies have examined the potential of feeding concentrates containing fish oil or marine algae to enrich 20:5n-3 and 22:6n-3 in muscle of growing cattle and lambs. Despite extensive biohydrogenation in the rumen, changes in the abundance of long-chain PUFA in muscle reflects the FA profile of dietary marine lipid supplements. Even though fish oil can be used to lower the n-6 : n-3 ratio, increases in the PUFA : SFA are often marginal (0.10 to 0.15). Given that 20-carbon n-3 fatty acids are incorporated mainly into PL rather than TAG, it is possible to enrich these PUFA in muscle without increases in fatness per se.

## Feeding of Plant Derived Bioactive Compounds

Bioactive compounds in plants can be defined as secondary plant metabolites produced within the plants besides the primary biosynthetic and metabolic routes for compounds associated with growth and development of the plant and are regarded as products of biochemical "side tracks" in the plant cells. Some of the plants have been observed to decrease the cholesterol content and in turn increase the quality of meat. Rana *et al.* (2012) studied the effect of supplementation of polyphenol rich *Terminalia cherbula* plant extract on FA composition of rumen fluid, plasma, intramuscular fat and A9- desaturase activity in *L. dorsi* muscle of cross bred kids. MUFA and PUFA content in muscle enhanced by 25 and 35 per cent, respectively, while the SFA content reduced by 20 per cent. A-9 desaturase activity increased by 47 per cent thereby increasing the total CLA content (58.73 per cent) in muscle which ultimately improved the meat quality. Supplementation of diet with plants containing bioactive compounds that affect bacteria (convert precursor of CLA to stearate) involved in rumen biohydrogenation is another useful strategy.

## Conjugated Fatty Acids

There has also been much recent research aimed at increasing the conjugated linoleic acid (CLA) concentration in milk fat because of its potentially powerful anticancer effect. Although ruminant foods contain numerous positional and geometric isomers with a conjugated bond system cis-9, trans-11 is the major isomer formed by endogenous synthesis via the action of stearoyl-CoA desaturase on trans-11, 18:1 (trans vaccenic acid) or during the biohydrogentaion of LA to stearic acid by *Butyrivibrio fibrisolvens* and other rumen bacteria. A number of nutritional strategies involving extended grazing, lipid supplementation have been developed to enhance CLA concentrations in milk. Concentrations of CLA are higher in milk fat from cows offered fresh forages as compared with conserved forages, can be enhanced using whole oilseeds or oil supplements in the cow's diet.

Fish oil increases the CLA content of milk fat more effectively than plant oils and these responses can be further enhanced when fish oil is fed in combination with plant oil supplements. Studies with growing lambs and cattle have shown that dietary lipid supplements can be used to enrich cis-9, trans-11 CLA in muscle up to 2.40 g/100 g fatty acids, cattle diets supplemented with 60 g sunflower oil/kg diet dry matter cattle resulted in cis-9, trans-11 CLA content of 134mg/100 g muscle.

## Conclusion

Food products derived from ruminants are important source of nutrients in the diet. However, certain aspects of these foods particularly SFA, have led to concerns about the contributions of these foods to increased risk of CVD and metabolic syndrome. Alteration in the fatty acid composition of ruminant derived food products offers an opportunity to align the consumption of FA in human population with the existing public health policies without bringing about changes in the eating habits. Though, nutrition is the major factor influencing the FA composition the application of genomic tools combined with a more complete understanding of the molecular mechanisms underlying lipogenesis offer the opportunity to breed genetic resources inherently suited to the production of meat and milk containing lower proportions of saturates and higher concentration of unsaturated fatty acids. The role of animal nutrition in creating foods closer to optimum composition for long term human health has become an important aspect due to the diet conscious consumers, however, the production of such foods on a scale that will affect the national diets will require both political and financial incentives and major changes in the animal production industry.

## Chapter 14

# Food Safety and Quality: Heavy Metals and Pesticides

*R.K. Sharma, R.P.S. Baghel, K. Shraman, Vidhi Gautam, Sunil Nayak and Ankur Khare*

*Department of Veterinary Pharmacology and Toxicology, College of Veterinary Science and Animal Husbandry, Nanaji Deshmukh Veterinary Science University, Jabalpur, Madhya Pradesh*

Food safety is a scientific discipline describing handling, preparation, and storage of food in ways that prevent food-borne illness. The occurrence of two or more cases of a similar illnesses resulting from the ingestion of a common food is known as a food-borne disease outbreak. This includes a number of routines that should be followed to avoid potential health hazards. In this way food safety often overlaps with food defense to prevent harm to consumers. The tracks within this line of thought are safety between industry and the market and then between the market and the consumer. In considering industry to market practices, food safety considerations include the origins of food including the practices relating to food labeling, food hygiene, food additives and pesticide residues, as well as policies on biotechnology and food and guidelines for the management of governmental import and export inspection and certification systems for foods. In considering market to consumer practices, the usual thought is that food ought to be safe in the market and the concern is safe delivery and preparation of the food for the consumer.

## Food Contamination

Food contamination happens when food are corrupted with another substance.

It can happen In the process of production, transportation, packaging, storage, sales and cooking process. The contamination can be physical, chemical and biological.

## Physical Contamination

Physical contaminants (or foreign bodies') are objects such as hair, plant stalks or pieces of plastic, glass and metal. When the foreign object comes into the food, it is a physical contaminant. If the foreign objects are bacteria, the case will a physical and biological contamination.

## Chemical Contamination

Chemical contamination happens when food is contaminated with a natural or artificial chemical substance. Common sources of chemical contamination can include: pesticides, herbicides, veterinary drugs, contamination from environmental sources (water, air or soil pollution), cross-contamination during food processing, migration from food packaging materials, presence of natural toxins or use of unapproved food additives and adulterants.

## Biological Contamination

Biological contamination refers to food that has been contaminated by substances produced by living creatures, such as humans, rodents, pestsor microorganisms. This includes bacterial contamination, viral contamination or parasite contamination that's transferred through saliva, pest droppings, blood or faecal matter. Bacterial contamination is the most common cause of food poisoning worldwide. If an environment has high in starch or protein, water, oxygen, neutral PH level and temperature between 5°C and 60°C (danger zone), bacteria are likely to survive. All above mentioned contaminants affects food quality which ultimately affects health of all. Safe food is must for good health. Human health and animal health are interdependent and bound to the health of the ecosystems in which they exist. One Health is the integrative effort of multiple disciplines working locally, nationally, and globally to attain optimal health for people, animals, and the environment. Together, the three make up the One Health triad. The one health concept in ecototoxicological perspective has gain less attention. Animal illnesses have alerted the medical community to toxicological disasters often well in advance of the appearance of adverse health effects in humans (NRC, 1991). In 1956, an outbreak of unusual and severe neurological illness occurred in Minamata Bay, Japan. The etiology was ultimately determined to be ingestion of locally caught seafood containing extremely elevated concentrations of methylmercury. The most severely affected individuals were exposed in utero (through maternal consumption of affected fish during pregnancy). Environmental toxicology has evolved in recent decades from an amalgamation of various scientific disciplines including biology, toxicology, environmental chemistry, biochemistry, pharmacology, and ecology. The overall objective of environmental toxicology is to understand the impact of chemical pollutants on ecosystems, encompassing all levels of biological organization– from biochemical interactions in biological organisms to whole animals, populations, and ecosystems (Escher, 2001).

The study of Ecotoxicology stems from the recognition that:

- ✰ Human survival depends upon the well-being of other species and upon the availability of clean air, water and food.
- ✰ Anthropogenic chemicals as well as naturally occurring chemicals can have detrimental effects on living organisms and ecological processes.

Ecotoxicology is thus concerned with how environmental toxicants, through their interaction with humans, animals, and plants, influence the health and welfare of these organisms.

Ecotoxicants are a diverse group of substances that have two general properties: they are discharged into the environment and they have the potential to impact on ecosystem at relatively low concentrations (Bols *et al.,* 2001).

Ecotoxicants can be classified into following categories:

A. Heavy metals
B. Biocides and their by-products
C. Industrial organic chemicals
D. By-products of industrial processes and combustion
E. Pharamceuticals

## Heavy Metal

### Toxicity Arsenic

Arsenic is one of the most important heavy metals causing disquiet from both ecological and individual health standpoints.It has a semimetallic property, is prominently toxic and carcinogenic, and is extensively available in the form of oxides or sulfides or as a salt of iron, sodium, calcium, copper, *etc.* (Singh *et al.,* 2007). Arsenic is the twentieth most abundant element on earth and its inorganic forms such as arsenite and arsenate compounds are lethal to the environment and living creatures.

Drinking water may get contaminated by use of arsenical pesticides, natural mineral deposits or inappropriate disposal of arsenical chemicals. Arsenic is a protoplastic poison since it affects primarily the sulphydryl group of cells causing malfunctioning of cell respiration, cell enzymes and mitosis.

### Lead

Lead is a highly toxic metal whose widespread use has caused extensive environmental contamination and health problems in many parts of the world. The sources of lead exposure include mainly industrial processes, food and smoking, drinking water and domestic sources. The sources of lead were gasoline and house paint, which has been extended to lead bullets, plumbing pipes, pewter pitchers, storage batteries. lead is being released from vehicle exhausts. Some is taken up by plants, fixation to soil and flow into water bodies, hence human and animal exposure of lead in the general population is either due to food or drinking water. A plant with high lead concentration fastens the production of reactive oxygen species (ROS), causing lipid membrane damage that ultimately leads to damage of chlorophyll and photosynthetic processes and suppresses the overall growth of the plant (Najeeb *et al.*, 2014).

## Mercury

The metallic mercury is a naturally occurring metal. Mercury is very toxic and exceedingly bioaccumulative. Its presence adversely affects the marine environment and hence many studies are directed towards the distribution of mercury in water environment.

## Cadmium

Cadmium is the seventh most toxic heavy metal as per ATSDR ranking. It is a by-product of zinc production which humans or animals may get exposed to at work or in the environment. Once this metal gets absorbed by humans, it will accumulate inside the body throughout life. This metal was first used in World War I as a substitute for tin and in paint industries as a pigment. In today's scenario, it is also being used in rechargeable batteries, for special alloys production and also present in tobacco smoke. About three-fourths of cadmium is used in alkaline batteries as an electrode component, the remaining part is used in coatings, pigments and platings and as a plastic stabilizer.

## Chromium

Chromium is the seventh most abundant element on earth (Mohanty and Kumar Patra, 2013). Chromium occurs in several oxidation states in the environment ranging from $Cr^{2+}$ to $Cr^{6+}$. The most commonly occurring forms of Cr are trivalent- $Cr^{+3}$ and hexavalent- $Cr^{+6}$, with both states being toxic to animals, humans and plants (Mohanty and Kumar Patra, 2013).

## Aluminium

Aluminium is the third most abundant element found in the earth's crust (Gupta *et al.*, 2013). Aluminium occurs naturally in the air, water and soil. Mining and processing of aluminium elevates its level in the environment.

## Iron

Iron is the second most abundant metal on the earth's crust. Iron occupies the 26$^{th}$ elemental position in the periodic table. Iron is a most crucial element for growth and survival of almost all living organisms (Valko *et al.*, 2005). It is one of the vital components of organisms like algae and of enzymes such as cytochromes and catalase, as well as of oxygen transporting proteins, such as hemoglobin and myoglobin. The concentration of dissolved iron in the deep ocean is normally 0.6 nM or 33.5 × $10^{-9}$ mg/L. In freshwater the concentration is very low with a detection level of 5 μg/L– ICP, whereas in groundwater the concentration of dissolved iron is very high with 20 mg/L (EPA, 1993).

## Nickel

Nickel is a naturally occurring metal that is sometimes present in food and water through environmental contamination, including as a result of human activity. Short-term (acute') exposure to nickel causes allergic reactions in some individuals, both by touch and also from ingestion in food or water. The results of animal studies also indicate possible reproductive and developmental effects from long-term (chronic') exposure to nickel.

## Pesticides

Pesticides, which are any substance intended to prevent or destroy pests, are used to protect food from bacteria, weeds, mold, insects and rodents. According to the Environmental Protection Agency, pesticides can be harmful to people, animals or the environment because they are designed to kill or harm living organisms. Because of this, pesticide residue on the foods you eat can have an effect on your health. Though the government regulates pesticide use, residues are still found in our food supply. The extensive application of pesticides is a common practice around the world. Although the production and marketing of certain pesticides harmful to humans have been banned, other products continue to be used, without knowing fully the negative impact that these compounds may have on ecosystems and public health.

**Herbicides**, also commonly known as **weedkillers**, are chemical substances used to control unwanted plants.

**Insecticides** are substances used to kill insects. Nearly all insecticides have the potential to significantly alter ecosystems; many are toxic to humans and/or animals; some become concentrated as they spread along the food chain.

An **insect growth regulator (IGR)** is a substance (chemical) that inhibits the life cycle of an insect. IGRs are typically used as insecticides to control populations of harmful insect pests such as cockroaches and fleas.

A **nematicide** is a type of chemical pesticide used to kill plant-parasitic nematodes. Nematicides have tended to be broad-spectrum toxicants possessing high volatility or other properties promoting migration through the soil.

Molluscicide, ***also known as*** *snail baits'* and **snail pellets**, are pesticides against molluscs, which are usually used in agriculture or gardening.

A **piscicide** is a chemical substance which is poisonous to fish. Examples of piscicides include rotenone, saponins, TFM, niclosamide and Antimycin A (Fintrol).

An **avicide** is any substance (normally, a chemical) which can be used to kill birds. Commonly used avicides include strychnine, DRC-1339 (3-chloro-4-

methylaniline hydrochloride, Starlicide) and CPTH (3-chloro-p-toluidine, the free base of Starlicide), and Avitrol (4-aminopyridine).

**Rodenticides**, colloquially **rat poison**, are typically non-specific pest control chemicals made and sold for the purpose of killing rodents.

Besides being directly toxic to the mammals that ingest them, including dogs, cats, and humans, many rodenticides present a secondary poisoning risk to animals that hunt or scavenge the dead corpses of rats.

A **bactericide** or **bacteriocide**, sometimes abbreviated **Bcidal**, is a substance that kills bacteria. Bactericides are disinfectants, antiseptics, or antibiotics.

**An insect repellent** (also commonly called "**bug spray**") is a substance applied to skin, clothing, or other surfaces which discourages insects(and arthropods in general) from landing or climbing on that surface.

**An antimicrobial** is an agent that kills microorganisms or stops their growth. Antimicrobial medicines can be grouped according to the microorganisms they act primarily against. For example, antibiotics are used against bacteria and anti- fungals are used against fungi. They can also be classified according to their function. Agents that kill microbes are called microbicidal, while those that merely inhibit their growth are called biostatic. The use of antimicrobial medicines to treat infection is known as antimicrobial chemotherapy, while the use of antimicrobial medicines to prevent infection is known as antimicrobial prophylaxis.

**Disinfectants** are antimicrobial agents that are applied to the surface of non-living objects to destroy microorganisms that are living on the objects. Disinfection does not necessarily kill all microorganisms, especially resistant bacterial sporesSanitizers are substances that simultaneously clean and disinfect.

## Conclusions

In considering industry to market practices, food safety considerations include the origins of food including the practices relating to food labeling, food hygiene, food additives and pesticide residues, as well as policies on biotechnology and food and guidelines for the management of governmental import and export inspection and certification systems for foods. In considering market to consumer practices, the usual thought is that food ought to be safe in the market and the concern is safe delivery and preparation of the food for the consumer.Heavy metals can be toxic for humans when they are not metabolized by the body and accumulate in the soft tissues. Depending on the heavy metal in question, toxicity can occur at levels just above naturally occurring background levels, meaning that consumption of food with a high heavy metal concentration can cause acute or chronic poisoning. Poisoning can result in damaged or reduced mental and central nervous function as well as damage to blood composition, lungs, kidneys, liver, and other vital organs. Long-term exposure to heavy metals may result in slowly progressing physical, muscular, and neurological degenerative conditions as well as cancer. Evidence indicates that pesticides pose a risk to public health, so it is necessary to conduct more studies using different models and indicators to assess the potential risks to health and the ecosystem. Therefore, unintelligent use of pesticides has led to reduced connectivity (trophic interaction between organisms), loss of biodiversity, ecological imbalance and environmental stability decreased. Consequently, man, by the lack of rational use of pesticides, has been and is threatening the sustainability.

## REFERENCES

Bols, N. C., Brubacher, J. L., Ganassin, R. C. and Lee, L. E. J. (2001). Ecotoxicology and innate immunity in fish. *Developmental and Comparative Immunology*, **25**: 853-873.

Escher, B. (2001). Molecular Mechanisms in Aquatic Ecotoxicology: Specific and Non-specific Membrane Toxicity. *A Habilitation Thesis in Environmental Chemistry and Ecotoxicology, Zürich, ETH Zürich, Habilitationsschrift*

Gupta, N., Gaurav, S.S., Kumar, A. (2013). Molecular Basis of Aluminium Toxicity in Plants: A Review. *Am J of Plant Sci.*,**4**: 21–37.

Mohanty, M., Kumar, P. H. (2013). Effect of ionic and chelate assisted hexavalent chromium on mung bean seedlings. (Vigna Radiata l. Wilczek. Var k-851) during seedling growth. *JSPB.*, **9**(2): 232–241.

Najeeb, U., Ahmad, W., Zia, M.H., Malik, Z., Zhou, W. (2014). Enhancing the lead phytostabilization in wetland plant *Juncus effusus* L. through somaclonal manipulation and EDTA enrichment. *Arab J Chem.*, (in press).

NRC (U.S. National Research Council), (1991) Animals as sentinels of environmental health hazards. *National Academy Press, Washington,* DC

Singh, N., Kumar, D., Sahu, A. (2007). Arsenic in the environment: effects on human health and possible prevention. *J Environ Biol.*, **28**: 359–365.

Valko, M.M., Morris, H., Cronin, M.T.D. (2005). Metals, toxicity and oxidative stress. *Curr Med Chem.*, **12**(10): 1161–1208.

## Chapter 15

# Technologies for Enhancing Fodder Production and Utilization in India

*A.K. Mehta*

*AICRP on Forage Crops and Utilization,*
*J.N.K.V.V., Jabalpur, Madhya Pradesh*

The livestock sector is valued as one of the global drivers of agriculture having enormous potential for poverty reduction. In India, integration of agriculture and animal husbandry is unique on account of rich and diversified cultural environment. Our economy largely depends on agro based activities as it sustains 65 per cent of population, employs 56.7 per cent of work force, contributes 20 per cent of GDP and accounts for 12 per cent of exports. The livestock is an important component of agriculture, is expected to exceed 517 million, which is 15 per cent of world livestock population as against only 2 per cent of geographical area. It is obvious from livestock data that it is the only asset evenly distributed between small and large farmers. Livestock is more popular among the weaker sections of society as they can invest in this asset even with limited resources. The livestock for farmer is not only a source of milk, meat, food, draft power and manure but also a symbol of social status and security against distress.

In our country livestock is based on low input, low output production system which may be sustainable for poor farmers but is not efficient in biological and economical terms. Our cattle and buffalo produce less than 1000 litres per lactation as compared to 4500 litres in Europe, 7000 litres in USA and 10,000 litres in Israel, livestock are usually under fed in India owing to high cost of animal feed which amounts to 60 per cent of livestock product costs.

With ever increasing livestock population there is urgent need to meet the demand of increasing number of livestock and also enhance their productivity for which availability of feed resources have to be increased. India has 15 per cent of world cattle population and due to ever increasing population pressure of human, cultivable land is being used mainly for food and cash crops. Thus, there is little scope of having good and quality cultivable land available for fodder production, until milk production becomes remunerative to the farmers as compared to other field crops. (DAHD, 2012).

Also, urbanization has brought a marked shift in feeding habits of people towards milk, meat and eggs with the consequential increase in demand of livestock products. There is no shortcut to sustain livestock husbandry, without focusing the issues related to the development of fodder and feed resources in the country. At present, the country faces a net deficit of 35.66 per cent green fodder, 10.95 per cent dry crop residues and 44 per cent concentrate feed ingredients. The demand will reach to 1012 million tonnes of green fodder and 631 million tonnes of dry forage by the year 2050 (IGFRI, Vision 2050). At the current level of growth in forage resources, there will be 18.4 per cent deficit in green fodder and 13.2 per cent deficit in dry fodder in the year 2050. To meet out the deficit, green forage supply has to grow at 1.69 per cent annually (IGFRI, Vision, 2050).

Therefore, it is very essential to increase the production and availability of fodder. This will help in increasing the productivity and profitability of livestock.

## Livestock and Forage Scenario in India and State

**Table 15.1. Animal Population of India and Madhya Pradesh**

| *Sl.No.* | *Species* | *Population (Million)** | |
|---|---|---|---|
| | | *India* | *M.P.* |
| 1. | Cattle | 190.0 | 10.15 |
| 2. | Buffalo | 108.7 | 9.47 |
| 3. | Sheep | 65.06 | 0.32 |
| 4. | Goat | 135.17 | 8.01 |
| 5. | Other animals | 18.17 | 8.37 |
| | **Total** | **517.1** | **36.32** |

*Economic survey, GoI 2017-18.

**Table 15.2. Fodder Requirement Availability and Deficit (Million Tonnes)**

| *Feed* | *Requirement (MT)* | | *Availability (MT)* | | *Deficit (per cent)* | |
|---|---|---|---|---|---|---|
| | *India** | *M.P.*** | *India* | *M.P.* | *India* | *M.P.* |
| Green fodder | 816.83 | 19.95 | 525.51 | 11.65 | 35.66 | 42.23 |
| Dry fodder | 508.99 | 37.41 | 453.28 | 24.30 | 10.95 | 35.04 |
| Concentrate | 139 | 3.19 | 78.2 | 3.74 | 43.74 | (+)14.7 |

*Draft IGFRI Vision 2050 document; **Prasad KVS, NABARD Souvenir National group Meet (*Kharif*-2015) p. 18.

## Crop Improvement

See Table 15.3

## Agro Techniques Developed

### For Irrigated Condition

Growing crop sequence of jowar+cowpea in kharif, berseem+sarson in rabi and maize+cowpea in summer for getting maximum tonnage of green fodder (1763 q $ha^{-1}$ $year^{-1}$) and net monetary returns of Rs. 57443 $ha^{-1}$ $year^{-1}$. Per day productivity (4.83 q $ha^{-1}$) of green fodder is also higher under this crop sequence as compared to other crop sequences.

### For Rainfed Condition

In rainfed areas, practice of introducing sorghum for fodder production as an inter crop with pigeonpea under 1:2 row proportion sown at 25 cm apart produced an additional sorghum green fodder yield of 537 q $ha^{-1}$ besides 12.7 q $ha^{-1}$ seed yield of pigeonpea.

### For Utera Condition

Relay sowing of berseem in standing crop of paddy at 15 days prior to its harvesting by using 40 kg seed $ha^{-1}$ not only saves the time and cost of field preparation but also increases the duration of fodder supply without compromising the production and profit.

### Forage Production Potential of Maize Grown for Baby Corn and Green Cob in Peri Urban Areas

The sequence maize (BC) + cowpea (fodder) – berseem – maize (BC) + cowpea (fodder) gave significantly higher net return of Rs. 110056/ha/year than other crop sequence and was closely followed by maize (green cob) + cowpea (fodder) – berseem – maize (green cob)+ cowpea (fodder). Fodder equivalent yield of cropping sequence maize (BC) + cowpea (fodder) – berseem – maize (BC)+ cowpea (fodder) was also maximum *i.e.* 2298.9 q/ha/yr.

**Table 15.3**

| Sl. No. | *Name of Crop* | *Name of Variety* | *Year of Release/ Notification* | *Breeding Institution* | *Adaptability (Region/area)* | *GFY (q/ ha)* | *Specific Characteristics* |
|---|---|---|---|---|---|---|---|
| | | | | **Kharif Crops** | | | |
| 1. | **Sorghum (*Sorghum bicolor* L.)** | SSG 59-3 | 1977 | CCS HAU Hisar | All Sorghum growing area | 700-750 | plants tall and profuse tillering with quick growth. tolerant to drought and water logging |
| | | M.P.Chari | 1978 | JNKVV, Jabalpur | UP, MP., Haryana and Punjab | 375-400 | Good for double cut under rain fed situation |
| | | Haryana Chari-308 (HC-308) | 1996 | CCS HAU, Hisar | All sorghum growing areas | 400-440 | plants tall with sweet stem, leaves long and broad |
| | | Pant chari 4 | 2000 | G.B.P.U.A.&T., Pantnagar | All Sorghum growing area | 400–450 | plants tall purple pigmented with dark green leave |
| | | COFS- 29 | 2001 | TNAU Coimbatore | All sorghum growing areas | 800-1000 | It gives 5–6 cuts in one year at 60 days intervals |
| | | Pant chari 5 | 2006 | G.B.P.U.A.&T., Pantnagar | All Sorghum growing area | 800–1000 | Plants tall, erect stem sweet and juicy |
| 2. | **Pearl millet (*Pennisetum americanum* L.)** | Giant Bajra | 1985 | M.P.K.V. Rahuri (Maharastra) | All Pearl millet growing areas | 500-600 | High GFY, leafy Moderately resistance to downey mildew and ergot disease |
| | | Raj Bajra Chari 2 | 1990 | RAU Bikaner Rajasthan | All Pearl millet growing areas | 300-450 | High GFY, resistant to foliar diseases and insect-pests |
| | | BAIF-Bajra- 1 | 2008 | BAIF Urulikanchan | North West and Central Zone | 400-420 | Superior for forage yield(GFY and DMY) and CPY |
| | | JHPM 05 -2 | 2008 | IGFRI Jhansi | All zones except South zone | 400-450 | Superior for forage yield (GFY and DMY) and CPY |
| | | AFB-3 | 2011 | AAU, Anand | Haryana, Punjab and Rajasthan | 450-470 | Superior for green forage and dry matter yield |

| *Sl. No.* | *Name of Crop* | *Name of Variety* | *Year of Release/ Notification* | *Breeding Institution* | *Adaptability (Region/area)* | *GFY (q/ ha)* | *Specific Characteristics* |
|---|---|---|---|---|---|---|---|
| 3. | **Maize (Fodder) *Zea Maize*** | African Tall | 1985 | M.P.K.V.Rah uri (Maharastra | All zones | 600-700 | Plants Tall, Stem thick, long leaves, resistance to foliar diseases and Stem borer |
| | | J 1006 | 1992 | PAU Ludhiana | All zones | 400-450 | Plants Tall, higher seed yield |
| | | Pratap Makka Chari | 2008 | MPUAT Udaipu | North West Zone | 450–500 | Superior for green fodder, dry matter and crude protein yield |
| 4. | **Cowpea (*Vigna unguiculata* L.)** | Bundel lobia 1 | 1992 | IGFRI Jhansi | Whole India | 300-320 | Good GFY,DMY Tolerance to major pest and diseases |
| | | Bundel lobia 2 | 1994 | IGFRI Jhansi | Central India | 275-290 | Good GFY,DMY Tolerance to major pest and diseases |
| | | UPC -625 | 2008 | GBPUT Pantnagar | North West, Central and North East Zone. | 350-375 | Superior for GFY,DMY and CPY. Resistant to mosaic, leaf spot |
| | | UPC -628 | 2009 | GBPUT Pantnagar | North West, Central and North East Zone. | 280-300 | Tolerance to major pest and diseases |
| 5. | **Rice bean (*Vigna umbellata* T.)** | Bidhan -1 (NC) | 2000 | BCKV Kalyani, W.B. | All rice bean growing areas | 275-300 | Superior for forage yield (GFY and DMY) and CPY |
| | | JRBJ-05-2 | 2011 | JNKVV Jabalpur | All rice bean growing areas | 300-325 | Superior for forage yield (GFY and DMY) and CPY |
| | | JRBJ-05-4 | 2016 | JNKVV Jabalpur | All rice bean growing areas | 240-260. | Early type, least susceptible to leaf blight, mosaic, and flea beetle |

| *Sl. No.* | *Name of Crop* | *Name of Variety* | *Year of Release/ Notification* | *Breeding Institution* | *Adaptability (Region/area)* | *GFY (q/ ha)* | *Specific Characteristics* |
|---|---|---|---|---|---|---|---|
| **Rabi Crops** | | | | | | | |
| 6. | **Oat (*Avena sativa* L.)** | Kent | 1978 | PAU Ludhiana | All Oats growing area of India | 500-525 | High GFY, bold seed type (SC and MC) |
| | | Bundel Jai- 822 | 1989 | IGFRI, Jhansi | All Oats growing area of India | 500-525 | Erect growth habit High GFY, (MC) |
| | | Bundel Jai- 851 | 1998 | IGFRI, Jhansi | All Oats growing area of India | 470-500 | High GFY and high regeneration potential(MC) |
| | | OS-346 | 2009 | CCSHAU Hisar | Central Zone | 480-500 | Superior in fodder and quality aspects (SC) |
| | | OS-337 | 2013 | CCSHAU Hisar | Central Zone | 480-500 | Moderately resistance to leaf blight |
| | | JO 1 | 2004 | JNKVV Jabalpur | Madhya Pradesh | 525-550 | Good seed setting ability after one cut(MC) |
| | | JO-2000-61 (JO2) | 2011 | JNKVV Jabalpur | Madhya Pradesh | 530-575 | High GFY and good seed yield (MC) |
| | | JO-03-91 | 2011 | JNKVV Jabalpur | Oats growing areas of central zone | 400-450 | Resistant to leaf blight, Sclerotium root rot, powdery mildew |
| | | JO-03-93 | 2015 | JNKVV Jabalpur | Oats growing areas of central zone | 475-500 | Resistant to leaf blight, Sclerotium root rot, powdery mildew |
| | | RO 11-1 | 2016 | MPKV ,Rahuri | All India except hill zone | 450-500 | Moderalely resistant to leaf blight, Sclerotium root rot, and less susceptale to aphids (SC) |
| | | JO 04-315 (JO-5) | 2016 | JNKVV Jabalpur | Madhya Pradesh | 575-600 | least susceptible against leaf blight, Aphids/tiller and Leaf defoliator (MC) |

| *Sl. No.* | *Name of Crop* | *Name of Variety* | *Year of Release/ Notification* | *Breeding Institution* | *Adaptability (Region/area)* | *GFY (q/ ha)* | *Specific Characteristics* |
|---|---|---|---|---|---|---|---|
| 7. | **Berseem (*Trifolium alexandrinum* L.)** | Mescavi | 1978 | CCSHAU Hisar | All India | 620-650 | High GFY,Wider adaptable |
| | | JB1 | 1979 | JNKVV Jabalpur | All India | 800-850 | Good for fodder and seed yield, Wider adaptable |
| | | Wardan | 1982 | IGFRI Jhansi | All India | 600-650 | High GFY |
| | | JB 5 | 2004 | JNKVV Jabalpur | Madhya Pradesh | 850-900 | Good seed setting ability. |
| 8. | **Lucerne (*Medicago sativa* L.)** | Anand Lucerne 2 | 1984 | AAU, Anand | All India | 600-650 | High GFY |
| | | Anand Lucerne 3 | 2009 | AAU, Anand | All India | 700-750 | High GFY |
| | | Anand Lucerne 4 | 2009 | AAU, Anand | North weast zone of India | 800-900 | High GFY |

**Effect of Planting Methods and Forage Crop Combinations on Fodder Productivity through Moisture Conservation**

- The combination of *Dichanthium annulatum* + *Desmanthus virgatus* planted with ridge and furrow method gave highest green fodder (511.0/ha/yr), dry matter (166.2/ha/yr) and crude protein yield (17.1 q/ha), it was closely followed by *Cenchrus ciliaris* + *Desmanthus virgatus* with ridge and furrow method, which obtained 432.4, 143.0 and 16.0 q/ha of green fodder, dry matter and crude protein yield, respectively.

## Future Thrust

- Collection, evaluation and maintenance of genetic resource of forage crops for genetic improvement as per mandate.
- Identification/development of genotype(s) for forage crops suitable during lean period.
- Development of multicut, dual purpose and disease resistance types in oat.
- To evolve dual purpose lines having high fodder tonnage along with good seed setting in berseem.
- Development suitable package of practices for improved varieties to maximize Productivity with minimum input.
- Identification of suitable fodder crop sequence for rain-fed situations.
- Enhance breeder seed production of mandate forage crops.
- Transfer of technology through KVK's and regional research stations.
- Human resource development through training of kisan mitra, REO's and extension workers by networking and capacity building.

## REFERENCES

Department of Animal Husbandry, Dairying and Fisheries, Ministry of Agriculture (DAHD). (2012). Annual report (2011-12). *Government of India, New Delhi.*

Economic survey. (2017). Government of India (website).

Vision 2050 IGFRI Perspective Plan. (2011). *Indian Grassland and Fodder Research Institute, Jhansi (U.P).*

Chapter 16

# Nutritional Approaches in the Control of Gastrointestinal Parasitism

*P.D. Juyal*

*Vice Chancellor,*
*Nanaji Deshmukh Veterinary Science University, Jabalpur, Madhya Pradesh*

## Introduction

Small ruminants have been the back bone of economy of rural landless farmers. The health status and subsequently the productivity of animals are often affected by the everlasting problem of parasitism. Parasitism may be of clinical and subclinical forms. Clinical form is often detected and treated by chemical anthelmintic; however, subclinical form remains undetected and imparts a significant loss in productivity in terms of meat, milk and wool. Subclinical forms first reduces the feed intake and resulting in reduction in productivity. Up to 6-30 per cent decline in feed and 40 per cent decline in live body weight gain have been recorded in lambs during subclinical helminthic infections (Poppi *et al.,* 1990). Chemotherapy with use of various anthelmintic has been the mainstay to control the parasitism. However, continuous development of resistant strains of parasites against these anthelmintic has become a new challenge in controlling the parasitism. Apart from this, residue in animal products and cost of these anthelmintic has been the added concern to chemical anthelmintic. Various alternative control strategies like grazing management, nutritional management, biological control, genetic control, vaccination *etc.* are being tried but none of them are showing desirable outcome individually. Out of them, nutritional management sounds good as the diet rich in protein, fibres, minerals, vitamins *etc.* keeps animal healthy and productive apart from discouraging the establishment of parasites in its gastrointestinal tract and helping in repairing the damage/deficiency caused by the parasites if any. So, the demand of hour is to exploit the nutrition-parasite interaction as an alternative approach to control parasitism as well as to satisfy the consumer's demand of safe residue free animal products.

## Pathophysiology due to Gastrointestinal Parasitism

The degree of influence of parasites on their hosts physiology/metabolism is depends upon the intensity of infection, invasive power and virulence of parasite, degree of adaptation between host and parasites, reproductive potential and tendency of release of toxic products and location of parasite in the host body. Apart from these, the various extrinsic and intrinsic factors inside and outside of their host such as age and breed of host, the level of nutrition, physiological and immune status of the host, concurrent infection, inclement weather (extreme weather), the level of hygiene, tolerance power of host *etc.* also influence the pathogenicity of parasites. The pathogenicity may be mild, moderate, highly pathogenic or even fatal.

Ruminants are generally parasitized by variety of pathogenic species of helminths. These species are associated with their specific locations within the host's gastrointestinal tract. The principal locations are the abomasum (*Haemonchus, Ostertegia etc.*), small intestine (*Trichostrongylus, Cooperia, Bunostomum etc.*), large intestine (*Oesophagostomum, Chabertia etc.*) and liver (*Fasciola*).

Before going into the detailed pathogenicity of parasites, let's understand the resistance and resilience of host to parasitic infection. The concept of resistance and resilience of the host emerged to describe the ability of host to withstand parasitic challenge. Resistance is the ability of the host by which it prevents or limits the establishment or development of parasite. Breed of host, plane of nutrition, previous exposure and innate immunity determine the degree of resistance of animals. On the other hand resilience is defined as the ability of the host to maintain reasonable level of production in the face of a parasitic infection.

The pathophysiological condition of host during parasitic infection is either by consumption of the digested food material or feeding upon various forms of host's tissue by parasites, consequently resulting in metabolic disorders and pathophysiological conditions that are not possible to cover up with any sort of nutritional supplements until the causative organism are dislodged and evacuated from the animal's body. Having said that the nutritional status of animal plays important role in influencing the establishment, fecundity and rejection of parasite population, however, it cannot replace the other control strategic measures like management, chemotherapy and prophylaxis in restoring the animal health and productivity. Therefore, the level of nutrition influences the resistance and resilience of host to parasitic infection.

It has been frequently suggested that the nutritional status of the host can influence the pathogenesis of parasitic infections and it is usually accepted that well- nourished animals withstand parasitism better than those less adequately fed (Whitlock, 1949; Gibson, 1963).

Once the parasites get into the hosts body, it cause reduction in feed intake, impairment in food digestion, decrease in absorption and utilization of digested food due to increased peristaltic movement of gastrointestinal tract resulting in early passage of digested as well as undigested food, consume the digested food and host tissues, damage the gastrointestinal mucosa resulting in protein, electrolytes loss and impaired absorption.

## Gastrointestinal Parasitism and Feed Intake

Reduction in feed intake in parasitized animal could be immune stimulatory or allow the host to become more selective in their diet (Kyriazakis *et al.,* 1988). Depressed feed intake may primarily reflect the response to an imbalance of nutrients reaching to liver and peripheral tissues because of the priority sequestration of amino acids by gastrointestinal tract for its repair as well as for development and expression of local cell mediated response. In an experimental study Kyriazakis *et al.* (1994) observed that lambs were selective for higher protein diet on giving dietary choice. Further, rapid restoration of appetite following anthelmintic treatment suggests that nematodes themselves may influence appetite directly through secretion of cytokine- like molecules (Kyriazakis *et al.,* 1996).

## Gastrointestinal Parasitism and Digestion and Absorption

Intestinal parasites adversely affect the digestion and absorption of dietary nutrients and host metabolism which in turn, affect the host's immune system and its ability to fight infection. The deficiency of specific amino acids could be due to reduction in net absorption of non-ammonia nitrogen (Coop *et al.,* 1997), secretion of amino acid containing products in gastrointestinal tract like higher secretion of threonine in intestinal mucus (Neutra and Forstner, 1987) and incomplete reabsorption of these amino acids (Bang *et al.,* 1990).

The reduction in nutrient availability to infected animal through both reductions in feed intake and/or reduction in efficiency of absorbed nutrients depend upon the species of parasites and its location in the gastrointestinal tract.

## Gastrointestinal Parasitism and Protein Metabolism

A series of experiments over the past two decades has established the fact that all helminthic infections are responsible for loss of considerable quantities of host protein into the gastrointestinal tract. The proteins represent plasma and frequently erythrocytes, exfoliated epithelial cells and mucus. It is more difficult to quantify accurately the losses of epithelial cells and mucus but indirect evidences suggest that these losses are also substantial (Poppi *et al.,* 1981).

In the parasitized animals, protein deficiency occur due to leakage across damaged intestinal mucosa and diversion of protein from production to enhance immune response against worms and repair of damaged intestinal mucosa. The immune system seems to be in direct competition with other body tissues for nutrients. Therefore, for infected animals, withstanding parasite load, maintaining immunity and normal performance is directly related to a high protein intake. The cell-mediated responses are likely to be protein demanding (Mac Rae, 1993) particularly for sulphur containing amino acids. In addition to these, there is need to repair damaged tissues, maintain blood or plasma homeostasis and mount an immune response have been shown to increase protein utilisation in splanchnic tissue by 40 per cent (Yu *et al.*, 2000) and reduce the amount of protein available for tissue growth and other activities. The losses in to the gastrointestinal tracts may be substantial ranging from 20-125 g protein/day in *T. colubriformis* infected sheep (Poppi *et al.*, 1986) and in *Haemonchus contortus* infection they can represent as much as 10 per cent of the circulating blood volume/day (Parkins and Holmes, 1989). To maintain the body growth in infected animal, there is increase in protein requirement due to loss or diversion of endogenous nitrogen. In lambs infected with *T. colubriformis*, the requirement of amino acids was found to be increased by 33 per cent at the expense of peripheral tissues such as muscles (Yu *et al.*, 1998). Thus, in totality gastrointestinal nematodes, the livestock production by absorbing the host's blood and food, damaging the gastrointestinal tract epithelial layer, depressing the appetite, decreasing the digestion, reducing energy retention, increasing nitrogen losses, decreasing absorption of amino acids *etc.*

## Influence of Nutrition on Gastrointestinal Parasitism

Nutrition has got a major influence on the severity of parasitism and some influences on the extent of acquired immunity. Research has shown that increased dietary intake of metabolisable protein and energy and high quality pasture can directly promote the host resistance and host resilience to worm infection (Knox, 2000). The effect of improved nutrition will be more dramatic in infections of young, naive hosts, which result in substantial pathophysiological changes and damage or loss of host tissue, such as occur in gastrointestinal parasitism (Holmes, 1993). Improving host resistance and/or resilience to infection through nutritional management can be one component in an integrated worm management approaches. The improved nutrition will always increase host resilience. In lambs acquisition of immunity has a greater priority than growth while in adult animal expression of immunity has lower priority than reproductive efforts. By nutritional management the increase in resistance/resilience to worms has been seen.

## Influence of Protein on Gastrointestinal Parasitism

In the light of the pathophysiological changes associated with gastrointestinal parasitism and especially the central role played by endogenous protein losses, host - nutrition and especially dietary protein intake might be expected to influence the pathogenesis of such infections. However, a number of studies indicated that protein supplementation appears to be most effective in enhancing particular immune response associated with latter stages in the acquisition of host resistance (van Houtert *et al.*, 1995). Young growing animals are more susceptible to gastrointestinal nematodes than adult animals and often can't get enough protein from pasture. Animals in poor body condition have a poor immunity.

Young sheep infected with black scour worms and given extra protein were found to have 45 per cent less number of worms in small intestine compared to those of non- supplemented sheep (Bown *et al.,* 1991). The rise (3-fold) in mast cell proteases activity in abomasum was found to associate with decreased establishment of larvae in sheep provided high protein supplementation (Coop *et al.,* 1995). The parasite rejection can be antigenic in nature but may also involve processes such as mechanical or enzymatic damage inflicted by the host on larvae or adult parasites.

Reduced FEC in animals offered high protein diet further helps in reducing the pasture contamination rate and subsequent re-infection. Further, up to 50 per cent reduction in faecal egg count (FEC) and worm burden was observed following infusion of casein in abomasum of *T. colubriformis* infested sheep (Bown *et al.,* 1991). Higher FEC and greater clinical severity of haemonchosis has been observed in sheep on low protein diet compared to high protein diet (Preston and Allonby, 1978).

Strain and Stear (2001) observed that lambs on diet with additional protein had shorter adult *H. contortus* and produce significantly more antiparasitic IgA. The IgA mediated suppression of worm growth and fecundity was assigned a major protective mechanism in sheep. The adverse effect of haemonchosis on production were minimised by feeding extra dietary protein to the infested animal (Datta *et al.,* 1998). Lower FEC and higher Packed cell volume and growth rate was observed in *H. contortus* infested lambs supplemented with cotton seed cake as extra protein compared to those which were fed wheat bran (Amynalem *et al.,* 2002). Sheep on diet containing 3 per cent urea gained more weight, consumed more feed and grow more wool of high fibre diameter than their counterparts given no urea (Knox and Steal, 1999).

The *in-vivo* studies demonstrated that sheep with urea in their diet had lower FEC when infested with *H. contortus* and/or *T. colubriformis*, but there was no effect of urea on egg count of sheep infected with *Trichostrongylus* alone. In contrast, *Trichostrongylus* numbers on slaughter were reduced in sheep fed diet containing urea whereas *H. contortus* numbers were not affected.

## Influence of Energy on Gastrointestinal Parasitism

In an experimental study, Bown *et al.* (1991) attempted to separate the effects of protein and energy supply on the resilience of growing lambs to a trickle infection of *T. colubriformis*. Using infusions directly into the abomasum of either casein, iso-energenic amounts of glucose or saline/mineral equivalents in sheep fed chopped hay these authors were able to demonstrate that the intestinal infection induced a protein rather than an energy deficiency. The resilience of the lambs to infection was maintained by the protein but not by the energy supplementation. However, protein- energy deficiency is an important cause of defective T-cell function (Chandra, 1984) and T-cells have been shown to play pivotal role in mediating acquired resistance to haemonchosis in sheep (Gill *et al.,* 1993).

## Influence of Micronutrients on Gastrointestinal Parasitism

Less emphasis has been given to the effects of micronutrients such as minerals and vitamins on parasitism, although it is known that the immune system has specific requirements for certain micronutrients such as zinc (Bundy and Golden, 1987; Chandra, 1993). Coop and Field (1983) suggested that an increase in phosphorus supply (from 1.88 to 2.75 g kg–1 DM) decreases mean worm burdens (from 11 000 to 1300) in sheep infected with a trickle dose of *T. vitrinus* over 14 weeks. These relationships need further investigation, since the effect of P supplementation will be influenced by the degree of hypertrophy induced in the small intestine which results in impaired absorption of P in parasitized animals (Bown *et al.,* 1989; Poppi *et al.,* 1990).

Trace elements (copper, Bang *et al.,* 1990; molybdenum, Suttle *et al.,* 1992a, b; selenium, McDonald *et al.,* 1989) can influence host resistance to nematode infection. They may have a direct anthelmintic effect as well as influencing host metabolism and therefore the levels of supplementation and the host's mineral status will be important. For example, Bang *et al.* (1990) demonstrated that administration of copper oxide wire particles to young lambs reduced the establishment of the abomasal nematodes *H. contortus* and *O. circumcincta.* In contrast, there was no evidence of an increase in worm burdens in lambs which were hypocupraemic (Hucker and Yong, 1986).

## Conclusion

On the basis of present knowledge on nutrition-parasite interaction, it can be concluded that there is strong support for the idea that host nutrition can affect the degree of host expression to parasite infection. Further, our understanding will improve by the investigations that investigate which effectors of the immune response are affected by host nutrition, and by considering quantitatively the role of specific nutrients in this interaction.

## REFERENCES

Amynalem, H.,Tembely, S., Anindo, D.O., mukasa-Mugerwa, E., Rege, J.E.O., AlemuYami and Baker, R.L. (2002). Effects of breed and dietary protein supplementation on the response to gastrointestinal infections in Ethiopian sheep. *Small Ruminant Research,* **44**: 247-261.

Bang, K.S., Familton, A.S. and Sykes, A.R. (1990). Effect of copper oxide wire particle treatment on establishment of major gastrointestinal nematodes in lambs. *Research in Veterinary Science,* **49**: 132-137.

Bown, M.D., Poppi, D.P. and Sykes, A.R. (1991). The effect of post-ruminal infusion of protein and energy on the pathology of *Trichostrongylus colubriformis* infection and body composition in lambs. *Australian Journal of Agricultural Research*, **42**: 253-257.

Bown, M.D., Poppi, D.P., Sykes, A.R. (1989). The effects of a concurrent infection of *Trichostrongylus colubriformis* and *Ostertagia circumcincta* on calcium, phosphorus and magnesium transactions along the digestive tract of lambs. *Journal of Comparative Pathology,* **101**: 11–20.

Bundy, D.A.P. and Golden, M.H.N. (1987). The impact of host nutrition on gastrointestinal helminth populations. *Parasitology*, **95**: 623–635

Chandra, R.K. (1984). Parasitic infection, nutrition and immune response. *Federation Proceedings*, **43**: 251-255.

Chandra, R.K. (1993). Nutrition and the immune system. *Proceeding of the Nutrition Society*, **52**: 77–84.

Coop, R.L. and Field, A.C. (1983). Effect of phosphorus intake on growth rate, food intake and quality ofthe skeleton of growing lambs infected with the intestinal nematode *Trichostrongylus vitrinus. Research in Veterinary Science*, **35**: 175–181.

Coop, R.L., Huntley, J. F. and Smith, W. D. (1995). Effect of dietary protein supplementation on the development of immunity to *Ostertagia circumcincta* in growing lambs. *Research in Veterinary Science*, **59**: 24- 29.

Coop, R.L., Kyriazakis, I., Huntley, J.F., Jackson, E. and Jackson, F. (1997). The influence of protein and amino acids on the resilience of sheep to intestinal parasitism. Proceedingof 4th International Congress for Sheep Veterinarians, Armidale, NSW, Australia, pp. 196-198.

Datta, F.U., Nolan, J.V., Rowe, J.D. and Gray, G.D. (1998). Protein supplementation improves the performance of parasitised sheep fed a straw-based diet. *International Journal for Parasitology*, **28**: 1269-1278.

Gibson, T.E. (1963).The influence of nutrition on the relationships between gastrointestinal parasites and their hosts. *Proceedings of the Nutrition* Society, **22**: 15-20.

Gill, H.S., Watson, D.L. and Brandon, M.R. (1993). Monoclonal antibodies to CD+4 T cells abrogates genetic resistance to *Haemonchus contortus* in sheep. *Immunology*, **78**: 43-49.

Holmes, P.H. (1993). Interactions between parasites and animal nutrition: the veterinary consequences. *Proceeding of the Nutritional Society*, **52**: 113–120.

Hucker, D.A. and Yong, W.K. (1986). Effects of concurrent copper deficiency and gastro-intestinal nematodiasis on circulating copper and protein levels, liver copper and bodyweight in sheep. *Veterinary Parasitology*, **19**: 67– 76.

Knox, M.R. (2000). Nutritional approaches to nematode parasite control in sheep. *Feed Mix*, **8**: 12-15.

Knox, M.R. and Steel, J. W. (1999). The effects of urea supplementation on production and parasitological responses of sheep infected with *Haemonchus contortus* and *Trichostrongylus colubriformis. Veterinary Parasitology*, **83**: 123-135.

Kyriazakis, I., Anderson, D.H., Oldham, J.D., Coop, R.L. and Jackson, L.F. (1996). Long-term subclinical infection with *Trichostrongylus colubriformis*: Effects on food intake, diet selection and performance of growing lambs. *Veterinary Parasitology*, **61**: 297-313.

Kyriazakis, I., Oldham, J.D., Coop, R.L. and Jackson, F. (1994). The effect of subclinical intestinal nematode infection on the diet selection of growing sheep. *British Journal of Nutrition*, **72**: 665-667.

Kyriazakis, I., Tolkamp, B.J. and Hutching, M.R. (1998). Towards a functional explanation for the occurrence of anorexia during parasitic infection. *Animal Behaviour*, **56**: 265-274.

MacRae, J.C. (1993). Metabolic consequences of intestinal parasitism. *Proceedings of the Nutritional Society*, **52**: 121-130.

McDonald, J.W., Overend, D.J. and Paynter, D.I. (1989). Influence of selenium status in Merino weaners on resistance to trichostrongylid infection. *Research in Veterinary Science*, **47**: 319-322.

Neutra, M.R. and Forstner, J.M. (1987). Gastrointestinal mucus: synthesis, secretion and function. In: Physiology of the Gastrointestinal Tract (Ed. L R Johnson) Vol.2, IInd Edition, Raven Press, New York, pp 975-1009.

Parkins, J.J. and Holmes, P.H. (1989). Effects of gastrointestinal helminth parasites on ruminal nutrition. *Nutrition Research Review*, **2**: 227-246.

Poppi, D.P., MacRae, J.C.,Brewer, A. and Coop, R.L. (1986). Nitrogen transactions in the digestive tract of lambs exposed to the intestinal parasite *Trichostrongylus colubriformis. British Journal of Nutrition*, **55**: 593- 602.

Poppi, D.P., MacRae, J.C., Corrigall, W. and Coop, R.L. (1981). Nitrogen digestion in sheep infected with intestinal parasites. *Proceedings* of *the Nutrition Society*, **40**: 116A.

Poppi, D.P., Sykes, A.R. and Dynes, R.A. (1990). The effects of parasitism on host nutrition-the implications for nutrient manipulation. *Proceeding of New Zealand Society Animal Production*, **50**: 237-243.

Preston, J.M. and Allonby, E.W. (1978). The influence of breed on the susceptibility of sheep and goats to a single experimental infection with *Haemonchus contortus. Veterinary Record*, **103**: 509-512.

Strain, S.A.J. and Stear, M.J. (2001). The influence of protein supplementation on the immune response to *Haemonchus contortus. Parasite Immunology*, **23**: 527-531.

Suttle, N.F., Knox, D.P., Angus, K.W., Jackson, F., Coop, R.L. (1992a). Effects of dietary molybdenum on nematode and host during *Haemonchus contortus* infection in lambs. *Research in Veterinary Science*, **52**: 230– 235.

Suttle, N.F., Knox, D.P., Jackson, F., Coop, R.L. and Angus, K.W. (1992b). Effects of dietary molybdenum on nematode and host during *Trichostrongylus vitrinus* infection in lambs. *Research in Veterinary Science*, **52**: 224– 229.

Van Houtert, M.F.J., Barger, I.A. and Steel, J.W. (1995). Dietary protein for grazing sheep: Interaction with gastrointestinal parasites. *Veterinary Parasitology*, **60**: 283-295.

Whitlock, J.H. (1949). The relationship of nutrition to the development of Trichostrongylidoses. *Cornell Veterinarian*, **39**: 146-182.

Yu, F., Bruce, L.A., Calder, A.G., Milne, E., Coop, R.L., Jackson, F. and MacRae, J.C. (2000). Subclinical infection with the nematode *Trichostrongylus colubriformis* increases gastrointestinal tract leucine metabolism and reduce leucine availability to other tissues. *Journal of Animal Science*, **78**: 380-390.

Yu, F., Bruce, L.A., Coop, R.L. and MacRae, J.C. (1998). Leucine metabolism across the gastrointestinal tract of sheep infected with *Trichostrongylus colubriformis. Proceeding of British Society of Animal Science*, 1.

Chapter 17

# Precision Feeding: A Developing Countries Perspective for Sustainable Animal Production

*Sunil Nayak, R.P.S. Baghel and Ankur Khare*

*Department of Animal Nutrition,*
*College of Veterinary Science and Animal Husbandry,*
*Nanaji Deshmukh Veterinary Science University, Jabalpur, Madhya Pradesh*

## Introduction

Population growth is challenging for agricultural systems around the world because it means producing more food to support an increasing population in a more efficient manner within the constraints of available natural resources, without compromising the future of coming generations.

Ruminants reared in temperate areas are generally fed on good quality roughages and with high levels of concentrate supplementation. However in the tropics most ruminants are fed on low-quality roughages, agricultural crop-residues/and industrial by-products which contain a low level of fermentable carbohydrate and a low level of good-quality protein. To optimize the utilization of the available feed resources for dairy animals, it is necessary to make the digestive system of the cow as efficient as possible by ensuring optimum conditions for microbial growth in the rumen and to optimize production by balancing nutrients so that these are used as efficiently as possible for milk production utilizing the maximum genetic capacity of the cow.

Low productivity of livestock in developing countries is the result of the breed, poor feed base and low feed conversion efficiency. The efficiency of nutrient use is very low and over 75 per cent of the nutrients end up lost to the environment, and causing pollution through emissions of the greenhouse gas, nitrous oxide and ammonia to the atmosphere, plus losses of nitrates, phosphate and organic N and P compounds to water. There is always an oversupply of nutrients, of imbalances between nutrients, reducing the efficiency of nutrient use which substantially increases N and P pollution levels. The major priority is for improving the utilization of low digestibility forage by ruminants is by optimizing the availability of nutrients from fermentative digestion. The efficiency of partitioning of absorbed nutrients into product by supplementation with critical nutrients that bypass rumen fermentation to augment and balance the nutrients absorbed to those required for maintenance, growth or productive function. As the nutrients needed for different function differ in priority, supplementation strategies will need to vary according to climate, environment, management and production targets in any one location.

Livestock operations today are characterized by narrower profit margins than in the past, whereas the competition in the market has gradually increased. However, profitability from animal production will increasingly be affected by globalization of the trade in feed and livestock/poultry products and competition for natural resources. Feed cost alone accounts for 60-70 per cent of production cost in animal production systems. However, in the near future the major challenge will not only be to increase the feed efficiency of animals, but also to mitigate the impact of the livestock industry on the environment (Godfray *et al.*, 2010), especially in developing countries, where it is predicted that livestock production will continue to expand because agriculture is still a major source of income (McAllister *et al.*, 2011). Feeding costs and nutrient excretion are to be minimized for sustainable animal production. It has been shown that optimization of animal production for maximal economic return with minimal excretion can be achieved to a large extent by applying precision feeding techniques.

## Precision Feeding

Precision feeding is based on the fact that animals within a herd differ from each other in terms of age, weight and production potential and therefore each have different nutrient requirements. Precision feeding involves the use of feeding techniques that allow the right amount of feed with the right composition to be provided at the right time to each individual in the herd economically and reducing the enteric emission of methane, excretion of nitrogen (ammonia), phosphorus and other compounds into the environment without jeopardizing animal performance and to formulate rations that maintain animal health without use of antibiotics, hormones or other materials of public health concern.

The essential elements for precision feeding in livestock production systems are the:

- Proper evaluation of the nutritional potential of feed ingredients,
- The precise determination of nutrient requirements,
- Formulation of balanced diets that limit the amount of excess nutrients,
- Concomitant adjustment of the dietary supply and concentration of nutrients to match the evaluated requirements of each individual in the herd as per different physiological stage.

Nowadays, areas like development of various technologies for improving nutritional potential of feed ingredients, technologies for site specific delivery of nutrients, development of biosensors, machinery or methods for accurate assessment and monitoring of nutrient content or metabolic indicators and animal response, development of immunity enhancers and development of additives, alternatives to antibiotics or hormones or harmful ingredients are also being considered under precision nutrition as these improves profitability or increases acceptability of animal products.

## Proper Evaluation of the Nutritional Potential of Feed Ingredients

Energy, protein, minerals and vitamins are essential nutrients that need to be supplied to producing animals in required quantity and in palatable form. In order to reduce feeding costs and nutrient excretion, proper assessment of the composition of the feed ingredients and their nutritional potential is absolutely essential. The assessment of the nutritional potential of feed ingredients and animal requirements have progressed from a gross to a digestible basis, and then to an available or net basis, allows for the formulation of diets with nutrient levels that are closer to the animals' actual requirements. Many factors are affecting accurate estimation of nutritional potential of feed like reliable method for assay of bioavailability of nutrients, lack of knowledge about metabolic fate of nutrients *etc.* (Stein *et al.*, 2007). Effect of processing and addition of enzymes should also be considered in determining nutritional potential of feeds. Nevertheless, the precise evaluation of the nutritional potential of feed ingredients is essential prerequisite for precision feeding.

## The Precise Determination of Nutrient Requirements

The actual nutrient requirement depends on animal factors (production level, genetic potential, gender, age and body weight, and health status), environmental factors (ambient temperature and humidity, space allowance, number of stress factors, *etc.*), as well as on nutritional factors (nutrient composition and ratios, digestibility of nutrients and level of anti- nutritive factors). The nutrient requirement can be well established/estimated with mathematical models. Nutrient requirements may also vary according to specific production purpose or response criteria *e.g*, optimum growth, protein deposition, feed conversion ratio, even economical or environmental response. Generally, two methods are used to estimate the nutrient requirements of domestic producing animals: empirical (medium to long term feeding trial) and factorial. In the empirical method, nutrient requirements are those that either maximize or minimize one or several sets of performance parameters during a period of feeding trial. In the factorial method, however, daily requirements are estimated as the sum of the requirements for maintenance and production. In the factorial method, requirements are estimated for each nutrient or its precursor and take into account the efficiency with which each nutrient is used for each metabolic function. In the empirical method, input output relationship is used to estimate the optimal response to varying nutrient levels of a population of animals showing some degree of heterogeneity. In contrast, the factorial method estimates, for a unique animal at one specific growing/producing state, the requirements at zero production and those allowing maximal growth/production. The empirical method estimates optimal nutrient allowances from a population perspective, whereas the factorial method addresses the needs of one reference animal during a very short period.

Mechanistic mathematical models that implement the factorial approach are proposed because of the complexity of animal responses and the numerous factors modulating them and thus the optimal level of nutrients that will optimize production systems (Van Milgen *et al.*, 2008). The nutrient requirement can be well established/estimated with mathematical models. An example is given in Figure 17.1 showing how digestible lysine requirement of pigs with different genotype changes during the growing and fattening period. The simulated genotypes have the same average daily gain (762 g/d) and daily feed intake (2.24 kg/d); however, the growth curves of them differ gaining 758 vs. 766 g/d in growing (30–65 kg) and 812 vs. 700 g/d in fattening period (65–115 kg), respectively. The digestible lysine requirement certainly differs and the genotypes have to be fed differently according to the dynamics of their growth otherwise the genetic potential cannot be realized and likely the slaughter quality is deteriorated. The advantage of using such models instead of table values is that the model can predict the nutrient requirement at any time point and not only in certain time period and thus the number of phases used during the pig production is a professional decision supported by well predicted data.

In order to be able to adjust the daily nutrition to the actual requirement of livestock the animals has to be checked by real-time body weight control. The body weight can be determined daily by a weighing adapter or by body shape analyser (Banhazi *et al.*, 2009). All the factors that influence production and therefore nutrient requirement should be controlled. In precision livestock farming the technology and housing conditions are optimized, however, if it is needed the nutrient supply can also be adjusted according to the changed environmental factors. The health and wellbeing control (behaviour and sound analysis, collecting physiological parameters like deep body temperature, respiratory rates) is also very useful; in case of confirming any disorder the problem can be fixed immediately.

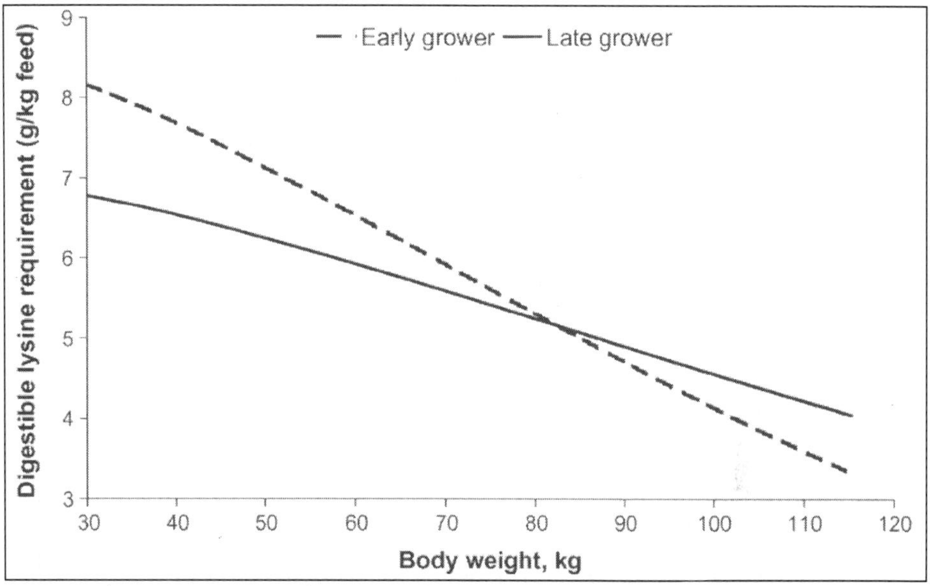


**Figure 17.1. Simulated Digestible Lysine Requirements for Two Pigs having same Average Daily Gain and Feed Intake but different Shapes of Growth Curve (Van Milgen *et al.*, 2008).**

## Formulation of Balanced Diets that limit the Amount of Excess Nutrients

Precision feeding is an attempt to feed as close to the exact requirement as possible on those nutrients that are expensive like amino acids or may have other detrimental effects when fed in excess like environmental pollution. It is also of providing available nutrients required by livestock for milk, meat and egg production, while reducing the quantity of the nutrients, especially nitrogen and phosphorous, excreted in droppings by minimizing the overfeeding of these and other nutrients. The long term benefits include the potential for lower feed cost, increased efficiency and reduced excretion of waste products. The potential drawback is that we may have slight reduction in growth rate or production performance as we feed closer to the true requirement. The nutrients those are of significant cost to the livestock industry consist of energy, protein/amino acids and phosphorus which are the three potential money savers that could be modified. Precision feeding is needed to minimize excess N and P.

The lactating cows should be fed according to their requirements based on the milk production ensuring optimum production with minimum excess N loss by optimizing the amount of rumen degraded protein and rumen un-degraded protein. For optimizing microbial protein production is to supply the rumen with fermentable carbohydrates, which stimulate microbial growth, along with N sources that meet microbial N requirements.

## Reduction of Nutrient Excretion by Increasing Efficiency of Utilization

To optimize the utilization of the available feed resources for animals, it is necessary to make the digestive system of the animal (ruminants) as efficient as possible by ensuring optimum conditions for microbial growth in the rumen and to optimize production by balancing nutrients so that these are used as efficiently as possible for milk production utilizing the maximum genetic capacity. Low productivity of livestock in developing countries is the result of the breed, poor feed base and low feed conversion efficiency. The efficiency of nutrient use is very low and over 75 per cent of the nutrients end up lost to the environment, and causing pollution through emissions of the greenhouse gas, nitrous oxide and ammonia to the atmosphere, plus losses of nitrates, phosphate and organic N and P compounds to water. There is always an oversupply of nutrients, of imbalances between nutrients, reducing the efficiency of nutrient use which substantially increases N and P pollution levels. The major priority is for improving the utilization of low digestibility forage by ruminants is by optimizing the availability of nutrients from fermentative digestion. The efficiency of partitioning of absorbed nutrients into product by supplementation with critical nutrients that bypass rumen fermentation to augment and balance the nutrients absorbed to those required for maintenance, growth or productive function. As the nutrients needed for different function differ in priority, supplementation strategies will need to vary according to climate, environment, management and production targets in any one location.

Ruminant nitrogen excretion is a major source of environmental pollution (FAO 2006). Total ammonia emission from livestock in India was estimated to be 1705 Kg/year out of which 23.6 per cent was contributed by buffaloes while 56.1 per cent was contributed by cattle. Only 5-30 per cent of dietary nitrogen is retained in body in case of ruminants. Ruminal amino acid deamination robs amino acids from the animal (Nocek and Russell, 1988). Most of the amino acid nitrogen that enters the rumen (60-90 per cent) are deaminated and rates of ammonia production often exceed the needs of ammonia - utilizing microorganisms (Flachowsky and Lebzien, 2006) but when it is excess the ammonia is absorbed across the rumen wall and subsequently converted to urinary urea and it is excreted through urine and faces. It has been suggested that reducing CP level and supplementation of rumen protected protein or amino acids (Lys+Met+His) should improve protein utilization efficiency without affecting milk yield. Hosam *et al.* (2013) reported that supplementation of the 14 per cent CP diet with 25 g/head/d rumen protected methionine increased ($P<0.05$) milk yield, fat corrected milk, energy corrected milk, percentages of milk fat, total solids and casein as well as yields of milk fat and protein compared to those without or with 15 g/head/d rumen protected methionine. Socha *et al.* (2008) reported that there was slightly increase of milk production and milk protein by dairy cows in early and mid lactation with supplementation of RPM and Lys in basal ration.

Recently ruminant nutritionists has increased focus on decreasing ruminal protein degradation and ammoniagenesis by focusing on controlling activity of hyperammonia producing bacteria (Gano, 2013) because the hyper-ammonia-producing bacteria (HAB) are bacteria that can produce ammonia at a rapid rate (>300 nmol $NH_3$/mg cell protein/min). HAB have minimal ability to utilize sugars and majority of them are considered to form an amino acid-utilizing niche. HAB have been isolated in cattle, sheep, goats (Flythe and Andries, 2009). Although only present in low numbers inside the rumen, the concentration of ammonia they are capable of producing makes them quantitatively important.

There is conclusive scientific evidence that dairy animals with low residual feed intake (RFI) consume less feed at the same level of production as high RFI animal. In addition to reducing feed consumption, animal with low RFI produce less methane from enteric fermentation and also less manure relative to high RFI cattle, due to the fact they consume less feed. (Arthur and Herd, 2008). Selection for lower RFI can reduce feed intake by 10-12 per cent, 25-30 per cent reduction in methane production, 15-17 per cent reduction in manure N, P and K excretion. Animals identified as more feed efficient at early age remain efficient throughout life and also produce offspring with high feed efficiency (heritability 35-40 per cent). A 5 per cent improvement in feed efficiency is equivalent to 20 per cent improvement in growth rate in economic term.

## Reduction in Methane Emission from Ruminants

Monitoring feed intake is one of the main constraints both for precision feeding and for estimate methane emission. Dry matter intake, in fact, is the main factors affecting methane emission (Hristov *et al.*, 2013). Different approaches have been evaluated to reduce methane emission from rumen like feed processing, ration balancing, supplementation, and development of plant based feed additives to reduce methane emission. Natural plant products containing essential oils (EOs), saponins, or tannins have been widely evaluated as non-antibiotic feed additives to mitigate methane emission, suppress protein degradation in rumen, increase feed utilization efficiency and improve characteristics of rumen fermentation (Calsamiglia *et al.*, 2008). Different research labs have been successful in identifying plant based feed additives which can reduce methane emission effectively but limited data is available on possible adaptation/development of resistance of rumen microbes to such additives.

According to Knapp *et al.* (2014), in dairy cattle the mitigation of methane emission by controlling nutrition approach may be obtained (i) altering the rumen VFA production pattern (ii) altering rumen microbe populations and increasing the rumen passage rate of digesta (iii) optimising feeding in order to increase milk yield (dilution effect).

Feed efficiency explains large part of the variability in methane emission intensity (Thoma *et al.*, 2012). Moreover, feed efficiency was identified as one of the most important parameters controlling GHG-emissions intensity, acidification and eutrophication potential in cattle (Cederberg *et al.,* 2009). A recent study demonstrated that when both energy and protein efficiency were improved, land use, water use, and GHG emission reductions ranged from 23.4 to 35.5 per cent (White, 2016).

## Adjustment of Nutrient Supply to Match Requirements of Livestock

Due to individual variance the nutrient supply that is fulfill the requirement of the maximal growth of a herd is not exactly the optimum for each individual animal within the herd. Actually the differences in individual nutrient requirement increase with the degree of heterogeneity of the population, which is determined by genetic, environmental or management factors (Pomar *et al.,* 2003). Such a system allows a daily adjusted feeding pattern for individual animal, therefore the oversupply attributed to phase feeding can be avoided. In this way the excess nutrients are reduced to zero and the efficiency of production is maximal (Pomar *et al.,* 2011). However, determining and offering the optimal nutrient supply for individual animals at any circumstances is very complex in practice.

Feeding individual animals as per their nutrient need considering individual feed efficiency will maximize efficiency of nutrient utilization in a farm. But such a practice is feasible only in fully automatic feeding management systems being introduced in many western countries. Development of automatic and intelligent precision feeder based on precision feeding techniques to automatically provide daily tailored feeds to each animal in the population, estimating its nutrient requirements each day based on individual feed intake and body weight measurements are under progress in developed country.

## Precision Nutrition Strategy for Small Livestock Farmers

The small livestock farmers of developing countries have limited resources available for feeding to their ruminant livestock. The available basal feed resources are essentially low digestibility forages such as tropical pastures (both green and mature), straws and other crop residues and agricultural by-products which are generally low in protein. It is important to establish the requirements for supplements that will provide nutrients that will optimise the efficiency of utilisation of that basal feed resource. This necessitates supplementation of limiting nutrients to optimize rumen microbial growth like NPN, amino acids, minerals *etc.* Any further increases in production may be obtained by the use of supplements of protein, starch and lipids to provide nutrients for milk production above those obtained when the efficiency of utilisation of the basal feed has been optimised. These supplements should be processed and must by-pass the rumen and become available for digestion in the intestine and in this way provide the nutrients in exactly the correct balance for additional milk production.

## Other Emerging Areas of Innovation for Precision Feeding

Key drivers for further innovation in precision feeding are Nutrigenomics, sensors- and nanotechnology and information and communication technology (ICT).

### Nutrigenomics

The nutritional requirements of farm animals have traditionally been estimated based on direct end points of animal performance, such as feed intake, body weight gain, feed conversion ratio, digestibility and health status as indicators. More recently, indicators on cell and tissue level were introduced. As a result, amino acid catabolism and immune, oxidative and intestinal health status can be measured nowadays.

Nutrigenomic technologies, such as genomics (DNA level), transcriptomics (gene activity at mRNA level), proteomics (protein level), metabolomics (metabolite level) and epigenetics (phenotype and gene expression level caused by mechanisms other than changes in the underlying DNA sequence) enable to refine such measurements (Hendriks, 2009). The end result will be a precise determination of the nutrient requirement of an animal under the specific conditions. Gut microbial nutrigenomics may offer opportunities in microbiota management which is the key to gut health and its associated immune system. The intestinal microbiota in its totality is viewed as the first line of defence to pathogens, because of its competition with invading pathogens for space, cellular receptors and nutrients and their role in balancing the immune system (Smits *et al.,* 2009). Although many aspects need to be exploited, bacterial nutrigenomics is seen as a breakthrough technology. All these powerful genomics tools will undoubtedly revolutionize the way we feed pigs and poultry and manage their production systems.

### Genomics

Some of the genomics technology, have already been applied in plant breeding. Most of the transgenic varieties grown today are known as first generation transgenics, because the transgenic trait provides benefits to crop farmers. Plants of the second generation may benefit the feed producers and farmers with nutritional enhancement, enzyme activity, immune enhancers or even natural antimicrobial substances.

### Fermentation

Another application of the omics' technologies is in industrial fermentation biotechnology. Industrial fermentation is the intentional use of fermentation by microorganisms, such as bacteria and fungi, to make products useful for humans or animals. Amino acids and enzymes are well known; both are crucial for optimization of performance of ruminants, pig and poultry. However, fermentation can also be used to improve raw materials. Digestibility of nutrients in general can be improved and the amino acid profile adapted closer to ideal patterns.

## Marker Technology

DNA-based markers affecting traits that are difficult to measure, such as meat quality, feed efficiency and disease resistance, will offer opportunities to improve product quality, increasing animal welfare, disease resistance and reducing environmental impact (Leakey *et al.,* 2009).

## Biosensors

A biosensor is an analytical device that converts a biological response into an electrical signal. The term biosensor' is often used to cover sensor devices used in order to determine the concentration of substances and other parameters of biological interest even where they do not utilise a biological system directly. There are many potential applications of biosensors of various types in animal production. In particular, the monitoring of macro- and micronutrients, additives, pathogens, contaminants and toxic metabolites in- and outside the animal may offer the possibility to fine tune performance in a well controlled environment (Luong *et al.,* 2008).

## Nanotechnology

Nanotechnology refers to an extremely dynamic field of research and application associated with particles of 1–100 nm in size (the size range of many molecules). Some particles of this size have peculiar physical and chemical properties, and it is such properties that nanotechnology seeks to exploit. Some food and nutrition products containing nanoscale additives are already commercially available, and nanotechnology is in widespread use in advanced agrichemicals and agrichemical application systems (Brunori *et al.,* 2008). Nanosized, multipurpose sensors are already being developed that can report on the physiological status of animals. Advances can be expected in drug delivery methods using nanotubes and other nanoparticles that can be precisely targeted. Nanoparticles may be able to induce more efficient utilization of nutrients by animals. One possible approach to animal waste management involves adding nanoparticles to manure to enhance biogas production from anaerobic digesters or to reduce odours (Scott, 2006). There are, however, considerable public concern regarding the possible human health and environmental impacts of nanoparticles and these risks will have to be addressed by risk assessment and regulation (Speiser, 2008).

## ICT

ICT consists of all technical means used to handle information and aid communication, including computer and network hardware as well as necessary software. ICT based automated feeding systems enable precision feeding leading to less spoilage of nutrients, and together with automated climate control will result in better animal health and welfare, and higher animal performance.

## Near-infrared Spectroscopy

Another application of ICT of relevance for animal feeding is near-infrared spectroscopy (NIRS). Over the past 30 years, NIRS has proved to be one of the most efficient and advanced tools for continuous monitoring and controlling of process and product quality in food and feed production. The accuracy of nutrient measurements and energy levels is increasing rapidly and even the detection of certain micronutrients, amino acids, undesirable substances and microorganisms *etc.* may be feasible.

## Conclusions

The dairy cattle are generally fed on diets with a margin of safety to minimize production risk especially in high yielding cows. The major focus has always been on maximizing production for better profits and now it's time to protect our environment by reducing the excretion of nutrients by a precision nutrition approach. The key factors are ration balancing, optimum use of protected amino acids, protected fat, good quality forages, proper ratio of RDP and UDP improving the efficiency of poor quality feed and crop management strategies.

## REFERENCES

Arthur, P.F. and Herd, R.M. (2008). Residual feed intake in beef cattle. *Revista Brasileira de Zootecnia* (*Brazilian Journal of Animal Science*), 37 (Special Supplement): 269-279.

Banhazi, T., Babinszky, L., Halas,V., Tscharke, M. and Lewis, B.(2009). Precision nutrition and smart farming developments for sustainable agriculture production. In: proceedings of the 14th *International Symposium on Animal Nutrition,* Kaposvár, Hungary, October 6, 2009. Kaposvár, University Press. 83–95.

Brunori, G., Rand, S. and Proost, J. (2008). Towards a conceptual framework for agricultural and rural inno-vation policies. IN-SIGHT-Project, IfLS Frankfurt/M.

Calsamiglia, S., Busquet, M., Cardozo, P.W., Castillejos, L. and Ferret, A. (2008). Essential oils as modifiers of rumen microbial fermentation. *Journal of Dairy Science,* 90: 2580-2595.

Cederberg, C., Sonnesson, U., Henriksson, M., Sund, V., and Davis, J. (2009). Greenhouse gas emissions from Swedish production of meat, milk and eggs 1990 and 2005 (SIK Report 793). Gothenberg, Sweden: Swedish Institute for Food and Biotechnology.

FAO (2006). Livestock's long shadow—environmental issues and options by Steinfeld H, Gerber P, Wassenaar T, Castel V, Rosales M. C Rome, DeHaan.

FAO (2011). World Livestock 2011 – Livestock in food security, FAO, Rome.

FAO (2016). The future of food and agriculture – Trends and challenges. Rome.

Available: http: //www.fao.org/3/a-i6583e.pdf

Flachowsky, G. and Lebzien, P.(2006). Possibilities for reduction of nitrogen (N) excretion from ruminants and the need for further research a review. *Landbauforschung Vo¨lkenrode* 56: 1930.

Flythe, M.D. and Andries, K. (2009). The effects of monensin on amino acid catabolizing bacteria isolated from the Boer goat rumen. *Small Ruminant Research*, 81: 178–181.

Gano, M. (2013). Amino acidfermenting bacteria from the rumen of dairy cattle enrichment, isolation, characterization, and interaction with Entodinium caudatum. Thesis. Graduate Program in Animal Sciences, pp. 1–128. The Ohio State University, USA.

Godfray, H.C.J., Beddington, J.R., Crute, I.R., Haddad, L., Lawrence, D., Muir, J.F., Pretty, J., Robinson, S., Thomas, S.M. and Toulmin, C. (2010). Food security: The challenge of feeding 9 billion people. *Science,* 327, 812-818.

Hendriks, A.T.W.M. (2009). Pretreatments to enhance the digestibility of lignocellulosic biomass. *Bioresource Technology*. 100 (1); 10-18.

Hosam, H.T., Saleh, I.A. and Mufeed, A. A. (2013). Effect of protected methionine supplementation on milk production and reproduction in first calf heifers. *Archiv Tierzucht*, 56(22): 225–236.

Hristov, A.N., Oh, J., Firkins, J.L. Dijkstra, J., Kebreab, E., Waghorn, G., Makkar, H.P.S., Adesogan, A.T., Yang, W., Lee, C. and Gerber, P.J. (2013). Special topics – Mitigation of methane and nitrous oxide emissions from animal operations: I. A review of enteric methane mitigation options. *Journal of Animal Science*, 91: 5045-5069.

Kearney, J. 2010. Review: Food consumption trends and drivers. Philosophical Transactions of the Royal Society B 365, 2793-2807.

Knapp, J.R., Laur, G.L. Vadas, P.A., Weiss, W.P. and Tricarico, J.M. 2014. Invited review: Enteric methane in dairy cattle production: Quantiying the opportunities and impact of reducing emissions. *Journal of Dairy Science*, 97: 3231-3261.

Knapp, J.R., Laur, G.L. Vadas, P.A., Weiss, W.P. and Tricarico, J.M. 2014. Invited review: Enteric methane in dairy cattle production: Quantiying the opportunities and impact of reducing emissions. *Journal of Dairy Science*, 97: 3231-3261.

Leakey, A.D.B., Ainsworth, E.A., Bernacchi, C.J., Rogers, A., Long, S.P. and Ort, D.R. 2009. Elevated $CO_2$ effects on plant carbon, nitrogen, and water relations: six important lessons from FACE. *Journal of Experimental Botany*, 60: 2859–2876.

Luong, J.H., Male, K.B. and Glennon, J.D. 2008. Biosensor technology: technology push versus market pull. *Biotechnol Adv*. 26(5): 492-500.

McAllister, T.A. (2011). Greenhouse gases in animal agriculture - Finding a balance between food production and emissions. *Animal Feed Science and Technology,* 166-167, 1-6.

Nocek, J. and Russell, J.B. 1988. Protein and carbohydrate as an integrated system. Relationship of ruminal availability to microbial contribution and milk production. *Journal of Dairy Science*, 71: 2070–2107.

Pomar, C., Hauschild, L., Zhang G.H., Pomar J. and Lovatto, P.A. 2011. Precision feeding can significantly reduce feeding cost and nutrient excretion in growing animals. In: modelling nutrient digestion and utilisation in farm animals Sauvant, D., Van Milgen, J., Faverdin, P., and Friggens, N. (eds.). Wageningen Academic publishers: 327–334.

Pomar, C., Kyriazakis, I., Emmans, G.C., Knap, P.W. 2003. Modeling stochasticity: dealing with populations rather than individual pigs. *Journal of Animal Science,* 81: 178–186.

Ray, P. P., J. Jarrett, and K. F. Knowlton. 2013. Effect of dietary phytate on phosphorus digestibility indairy cows. *Journal of Dairy Science*. 96: 1156-1163.

Scott, N. R. 2006. Impact of nanoscale technologies in animal management. The Netherlands: Wageningen Academic Publishers. WAAP Book of the Year 2006, 283–291.

Smits E.A., Quinn C.F., Tapken, W., Malagoli, M and Schiavon M. 2009. Physiological functions of beneficial elements. *Curr Opin Plant Biol*. 12 (3): 267-74.

Socha, M. T., C. G. Schwab, D. E. Putnam, N. L. Whitehouse, B. D. Garthwaite, and

G. A. Ducharme. 2008. Extent of methionine limitation in peak, early, and mid-lactation dairy cows. *Journal of Dairy Science,* 91: 1996–2010.

Speiser, B. 2008. Nano-particles in organic production? Issues and opinions. Paper presented at 16th IFOAM Organic World Congress, Modena, Italy, 18–20 June 2008.

Stein, H.H., Seve, B., Fuller, M.F., Moughan, P.G. and De Lange, C.F.M. 2007. Invited review: Amino acid bioavailability and digestibility in pig feed ingredients: terminology and application. *Journal of Animal Science*, 85: 172–180.

Steinfeld, H., Gerber, P., Wassenaar, T., Castel, V., Rosales, M. and de Haan, C. 2006. Livestock's Long Shadow: Environmental Issues and Options. Rome: Food and Agriculture Organization of the United Nations.

Thoma, G., Popp, J., Shonnard, D., Nutter, D., Matlock, M., Ulrich, R. 2012. Regional analysis of greenhouse gas emissions from US dairy farms: a cradle to farm-gate assessment of the American dairy industry circa 2008. *International Dairy Journal*.

Van Milgen, J., Valancogne, A., Dubois, S., Dourmad, J.Y., Sève B and Noblet, J. 2008. Inraporc: A model and decision support tool for the nutrition of growing pigs. *Animal Feed Science and Technology*, 143: 387–405.

White, R.R. 2016. Increasing energy and protein use efficiency improves opportunities to decrease land use, water use, and greenhouse gas emissions from dairy production. *Agricultural Systems*, 146: 20-29.

Chapter 18

# Management of Improved Rural Poultry Birds for Doubling Farmers Income

*J.K. Bhardwaj*

*Nanaji Deshmukh Veterinary Science University, Jabalpur, Madhya Pradesh*

Poultry sector plays a significant role in our country's GDP besides providing employment opportunities to significant percentage of population. Poultry production system in India as it exists today is characterized by simultanceous existence of the traditional extensive system of backyard production and modern intensive system of management. The later has eolved form the former and has organized it self into a vertically integrated and organized from during last 40 years. The modern industry has achieved an impressive growth during this short period and its accounts for about 65 per cent of total poultry meat and egg production in the country at present. The traditional system (backyard, semi-intensive) is gaining its importance day-by-day due to interest of consumers towards organic farming products and most important contribution of poultry is the rich protein it provides to the human diet. Several managemental factors influence the growth production performance and livability of chicken.

In the rural scenario poultry do not need any land, birds are easy to manage with these hardy birds managing themselves most of the time in a set pattern, returning faithfully home for the night and regularly laying eggs at home.

Village chickens play an integral role in small holder farming systems. The small holder chicken sector is traditionally based on extensive free range systems where the birds find most of their feed through scavenging. Small farming families land less labourers and people with income below the poverty line rear chickens with low inputs and harvests the benefits like egg and meat via scavenged feed resources. Chicken meat and egg provide a readily available, high quality source of protein, vitamins and micronutrients which are particularly essential for children, pregnant women and nursery mothers, thus helps to meet out the nutritional needs of the rural population. Village chickens are also active in pest control, provide manure feathers *etc.* are required for special festivals and are essential for many traditional ceremonies. Household sell chicken to generate cash. They are used to meet social, economic and cultural need of household.

Traditional poultry keeping in the backyard is still a potential source of live stock component among the tribal's and rural poor. It will continue, indefinitely as it is an important source of income generation to meet their urgent needs. Native chicken in rural and tribal areas constitute about 40 per cent of chicken population. However their average agg laying capacity is about 30-60 eggs annually and growth is slow (100 to 180 days to attain 1 kg live body weight). But desi eggs and meat fetch a much higher price than that from commercial poultry.

M.P is having 10 ten districts with between 25.50 per cent tribal population and five districts with more than 50 per cent tribal population. (Jhabua, Dhar, Darwani, Dindori (64.8 per cent) Mandla (57.23 per cent) As for as Madhya Pradesh is concerned the proportion of rural Poultry in nearly about 62 per cent of the total Poultry Population of the state Still majority of poultry birds are maintained under backyard/free range system in M.P. by the tribal's and rural Poultry farmers.

## Salient Features of Improved Coloured Bird

- ☆ It must have very attractive multi colour plumage pattern (brown, black, grey, mixed) and personality.
- ☆ Due to long shank, upright leanear appearance, strong body conformation move faster in free range for scavenging and also protect themselves from predators.
- ☆ It easily adapts the rural environments, so suitable in backyard and small scale poultry system.
- ☆ May Survive better in sub-optimal nutrition and management.
- ☆ Produce brown shell egg as deshi, not in bigger size (50 g) tasty as these birds are dependent on natural feed from the surrounding.
- ☆ Faster growth rate, male should attained 1 kg body weight in 9-10 weeks of age. Adult 20 weeks b. wt. from 1500 to 2200g in males and 1300 to 1700g in females.

- The female should mature on an average 165 days of age (intensive) and produce at least 3 times higher than the local native (45 eggs) in backyard and 4 times under semi intensive system of management.
- High suitability and adaptability under rural management system.
- It may be of dual purpose, egg type or meat type as per farmer preforance.

## Rearing and Management

### Breeding of Chicks

A newly hatched chicks has not developed the thermoregulatory mechanism fully and takes about 2 weeks to develop this mechanism and homeostasis. Therefore they cannot maintain the body temperature properly for the first weeks of life and may be subjected to the chilling, if not properly taken care of. Chicks need brooding during the initial 4-6 weeks of age to maintain the required body temperature. Artificial heat can be provided by bulbs, infra red bulbs, heat coil, brooders made of wooden/metal/locally available material. The brooding arrangement can be made either in floor or in cage as per available facilities. After cleaning, washing and disinfecting the brooder house, equipments, utensils close it until arrival of chicks. Spread the litter material 2-3 inches uniformly and spread news paper over litter for 3-4 days to prevent baby chicks for eating the litter. Arrange feeder, waterers, alternatively in cart wheel spokes like fashion and use chick guard to restrict movement of chicks so they remains near heat source. Provide three 60-70 cm linear chick feeders or 2-3 plastic tube feeders and two chick waterer (fountains) for each 100 baby chicks. After 4-6 weeks of age they can be let free for scavenging in the backyard surrounding the house. During the initial acclimatization, care needs to be taken to habituate them to reach the nest in the evening for night shelter which must have good ventilation, required light and protection from predators.

### Feeding

Balanced feed fortified with required minerals, vitamins, antimicrobial and anticoccidial should be fed ad- lib during first 4 weeks of age for optimum growth performance. The diet can be formulated using the locally available feed ingredients like broken rice, jowar, maize, ragi, bajra, korra *etc.* as energy source and soyabean, sunflower, ground nut cake as protein source. Chick ration which is available commercially can also be fed during initial 4 weeks of age. It is important to ensure easy access of feed to all the birds and offer feed daliy. These chicks need about 17 per cent protein and 2600 ME kcal/kg of feed in diet.

### Health Care

During initial brooding period (4 weeks age) the chicks of must be vaccinated against Marek's, Ranikhet and IBD diseases.

**Table 18.1. Vaccination Schedule**

| *Age (Days)* | *Name of Disease* | *Strain* | *Dosage* | *Route* |
|---|---|---|---|---|
| Day old | Marek`s Disease | HVT | 0.2 ml | S/c injection |
| 7-10 | Ranikhet | F1/B1 | one drop | I/N or I/O |
| 14 | Infectious Bursal disease | IBD Living mild | one drop | I/N or I/O |
| 28 | Ranikhet | Lasota | ------- | Drinking water. |
| 9-10 weeks | Ranikhet | $R_2B$ Mukteshwar | 0.5 ml. | I/M |

## Free Range Management

After 4 to 6 weeks age chicks can be let free during day time for scavenging in the backyard surroundings of the home to rear the chicks(10 and above) depending on the availability of natural feed in the area. During night they return in the house and are kept in night shelter.

Incase of dual purpose bird, the males can be sold at any time after attaining the suitable/minimum or market body weight. At 8 weeks of age males on an average generally attain 750g body weight in free range 860g in semi intensive and 1170g in intensive system of management. Whereas adult male attained 2300 to 2500g b.wt. under rural management condition depending on the availability of natural feed.

## Feeding

The general practices adopted by most of the tribes for rearing of local birds without provision of supplementary feeding however some farmers provid kitchen waste, grains or feedwaste, and what so over available waste material of feed and vegetable sources. Birds under free range easily pick up its food from the backyard once it learns to scavange in the feed. Additional feed supplementation requirement depends on the availability of scavange area vegetation, waste grain insects, grass seed *etc.* Birds generally fulfill their protein requirement through scavenging. It is also very fond of leafy vegetables like methi, palak, cholai, patharchata, leguminons leaf *etc.* Therefore grain supplementation (wheat, jowar, onaize, broun rice, korra always beneficial for better production performance. Resourceful farmers, of villages maintaining these birds only for meat purpose under intensive and semi-intensive system can provide commercial available broiler feed for better early growth. For laying of eggs single/community nest made up of wooden/earthen/ galvanized iron sheet with provision of hole should be used. One single nest is sufficient for 3-4 hens. For egg production to avoid breakage of egg supplementation of calcium sources like shell grit, stone grit, limestone, DCP powder. @ 3-4 g/bird/ day during laying phase is suggested.

## Housing

Housing is required for night shelter and protection from rains, predators.

About 1.5 to 2 Sq. ft. floor space is required per bird. Most of the farmers tribals maintaining these birds are resource poor farmer, having small holding. They provide basic housing as small Dadba to protect the birds from change of weather (heat, rain, cold, predators during night) such facility is created by using bamboo, waste wood of other available materials.Dadba must have the provision of small entry gate, bambaoo ventilation, wirer mash ventilation and roof covered with bamboo, local tiles, dry leaves or asbestos sheet may be used Periodic cleaning and spraying is needed form health point of view. Locally available materials like rice husks, ground nut hulls, wood shaving *etc.* can be used as bedding material and always keep it dry.

## Healthcare

A proper vaccination schedule as indicated above in table 1. should be followed to protect the birds against infectious diseases. The most important diseases that affect in free range is Ranikhet disease. So give vaccination against Ranikhet disease at 6 month interval by adopting cold chain. There is a possibility of parasitic infestation in birds so deworming at 2-3 month interval is required under free range condition. Periodically cleaning of Dadba, shed is necessary to protect form coccidiosis. Preventive dose of coccidiostat may be given between 4-6 weeks' age and curative dose during coccidiosis disease.

**Table 18.2. Performance of Narnadanidhi Birds (Dual purpose Colour Bird)**

**Suitable for Backyard, Rural and Tribal Areas Poultry Farming**

| *Economic Traits* | *Performance* | | | |
|---|---|---|---|---|
| Day old chick weight (g) | | | - | 38 |
| Body weight at 8wks of age (g) | Free range | | - | 605-765 |
| | Intensive | | - | 860- 1172 |
| Body weight at 20 wks age(g) | Free range | (M) | - | 1550 |
| | | (F) | - | 1314 |
| | Intensive | (M) | - | 2247 |
| | | (F) | - | 171 |
| Body weight 40 wks age (g) | Free range | (M) | - | 2310 |
| | | (F) | - | 1650 |
| | Intensive | (M) | - | 2650 |
| | | (F) | - | 1860 |
| Age at sexual maturity<br>Av.egg weight | Intensive | | - | 161<br>50.2g |
| Annual egg production | Free range | | - | 181 |
| | Intensive | | - | 223 |

## Chapter 19

# Functional Foods: A Boon to Human Health

*Ankur Khare, R.P.S. Baghel, Sunil Nayak and Pramod Sharma*

*Department of Animal Nutrition, College of Veterinary Science and Animal Husbandry, Nanaji Deshmukh Veterinary Science University, Jabalpur, Madhya Pradesh*

## Introduction

Let food be the medicine and medicine be the food- the tenet was embraced ~2500 years ago by Hippocrates, the father of medicine. In the recent years, a special attention has been paid in understanding the role of individual food ingredients as modulators of the body functions, which are responsible for maintaining and promoting health and welfare, or participating in prevention and reduction of risks of chronic diseases in the population. Scientists have begun to identify physiologically active components of foods from both plants and animals that have potential to reduce the risk for variety of chronic diseases (Hasler, 2002). Any food can be regarded as functional if it can be demonstrated to have beneficial effect on one or more target functions in the body or reduce disease risk besides basic nutrition (Bellisle *et al.,* 1998). According to Clydesdale, (1997), functional food has a physiological or psychological connotation beyond its traditional effect.

Functional properties of many traditional foods are being discovered, while new food products are being developed having beneficial components. Although the majority of physiologically active food components are of plant origin, animal products also have several substances with a potential role in health promotion. When farm animals are concerned for the production of functional foods it is primarily associated with the nutrition management, which is possible by either increasing or decreasing the ratio of biologically active components in their products. It is important that each animal category is given adequate feed, which will generate beneficial effects on the animal welfare and health, and indirectly also, on human health.

## Functional Foods from Plant Sources

Overwhelming evidence from epidemiological, *in vivo, in vitro,* and clinical trial data indicates that a plant-based diet can reduce the risk of chronic disease, particularly in cancer. In 1992, a review of 200 epidemiological studies (Block *et al.,* 1992) showed that cancer risk in people consuming diets high in fruits and vegetables was only one-half that in those consuming few of these foods. It is now clear that there are components in a plant-based diet other than traditional nutrients that can reduce cancer risk. Steinmetz and Potter (1991a) identified more than a dozen classes of these biologically active plant chemicals, now known as "phytochemicals."

### Oats

Oat products are a widely studied dietary source of the cholesterol-lowering soluble fiber beta-glucan. There is now significant scientific agreement that consumption of this particular plant food can reduce total and low density lipoprotein (LDL) cholesterol, thereby reducing the risk of coronary heart disease (CHD). The daily amount of oat bran or oatmeal consumed ranged from 34 g to 123 g. Quaker Oats determined that 3 g of b-glucan would be required to achieve a 5 per cent reduction in serum cholesterol, an amount equivalent to approximately 60 g of oatmeal or 40 g of oat bran (dry weight). Thus, a food bearing the health claim must contain 13 g of oat bran or 20 g oatmeal, and provide, without fortification, at least 1.0 g of b-glucan per serving.

### Soybean

The cholesterol-lowering effect of soybean is the most well-documented physiological effect. Studies found that the consumption of soybean protein resulted in significant reductions in total cholesterol (9.3 per cent), LDL cholesterol (12.9 per cent), and triglycerides (10.5 per cent), with a small but insignificant increase (2.4 per cent) in high density lipoprotein (HDL) cholesterol (Anderson *et al.,* 1995). Linear regression analysis indicated that the threshold level of soybean intake at which the effects on blood lipids became significant was 25 g.

Several classes of anticarcinogens have been identified in soybeans, including protease inhibitors, phytosterols, saponins, phenolic acids, phytic acid, and isoflavones (Messina and Barnes, 1991). Isoflavones (genistein and daidzein) are particularly noteworthy because soybeans are the only significant dietary source of these compounds. Isoflavones are heterocyclic phenols structurally similar to the estrogenic steroids. Because they are weak estrogens, isoflavones may act as antiestrogens by competing with the more potent, naturally-occurring endogenous estrogens (*e.g.*, 17b- estradiol) for binding to the estrogen receptor. This may explain why populations that consume significant amounts of soybean (*e.g.*, Southeast Asia) have reduced risk of estrogen-dependent cancer.

## Flaxseed

Among the major seed oils, flaxseed oil contains the most (57 per cent) of the omega-3 fatty acid, a-linolenic acid. Recent research, however, has focused more specifically on fiber-associated compounds known as lignans. The two primary mammalian lignans, enterodiol and its oxidation product, enterolactone, are formed in the intestinal tract by bacterial action on plant lignan precursors. Flaxseed is the richest source of mammalian lignan precursors (Thompson *et al.*, 1991). Because enterodiol and enterolactone are structurally similar to both naturally-occurring and synthetic estrogens, and have been shown to possess weakly estrogenic and antiestrogenic activities, they may play a role in the prevention of estrogen-dependent cancers. However, there is no epidemiological data and relatively few animal studies to support this hypothesis.

## Tomatoes

Tomatoes have received significant attention within the last three years because of interest in lycopene, the primary carotenoid found in this fruit and its role in cancer risk reduction.In a prospective cohort study of more than 47,000 men, those who consumed tomato products 10 or more times per week had less than one-half the risk of developing advanced prostate cancer (Giovannucci *et al.*, 1995). Interestingly, lycopene is the most abundant carotenoid in the prostate gland (Clinton *et al.*, 1996). Other cancers whose risk have been inversely associated with serum or tissue levels of lycopene include breast, digestive tract, cervix, bladder, and skin (Clinton, 1998) and possibly lung.

## Garlic

Garlic (*Allium sativum*) is likely the herb most widely quoted in the literature for medicinal properties (Nagourney, 1998). The purported health benefits of garlic are numerous, including cancer chemopreventive, antibiotic, anti-hypertensive, and cholesterol-lowering properties. Garlic components have been shown to inhibit tumorigenesis in several experimental models (Reuter *et al.*, 1996). However, additional reports have shown garlic to be ineffective. Inconclusive results are likely due to differences in the type of garlic compounds or preparations used by various investigators. Considerable variation in the quantity of organosulfur compounds available in fresh and commercially available garlic products has been demonstrated.

## Broccoli and other Cruciferous Vegetables

Epidemiological evidence has associated the frequent consumption of cruciferous vegetables with decreased cancer risk. In a recent review of 87 case-control studies, Verhoeven *et al.* (1996) demonstrated an inverse association between consumption of total brassica vegetables and cancer risk. The percentages of case-control studies showing an inverse association between consumption of cabbage, broccoli, cauliflower, and Brussels sprouts and cancer risk were 70, 56, 67, and 29 per cent, respectively. Anticarcinogenic properties of cruciferous vegetables is attributed to their relatively high content of glucosinolates.

## Citrus Fruits

Several epidemiological studies have shown that citrus fruits are protective against a variety of human cancers. Although oranges, lemons, limes, and grapefruits are a principal source of such important nutrients as vitamin C, folate, and fiber, Elegbede *et al.* (1993) have suggested that another component is responsible for the anticancer activity. Citrus fruits are particularly high in a class of phytochemicals known as the limonoids.

## Cranberry

Cranberry juice has been recognized as efficacious in the treatment of urinary tract infections since 1914, when benzoic acid-rich fruit caused acidification of the urine. Recent investigations have focused on the ability of cranberry juice to inhibit the adherence of Escherichia coli to uroepithelial cells (Schmidt and Sobota, 1988). This phenomenon has been attributed to two compounds: fructose and a nondialyzable polymeric compound. The latter compound, subsequently isolated from cranberry and blueberry juices (Ofek *et al.*, 1991), was found to inhibit adhesins present on the pili of the surface of certain pathogenic *E. coli.*

## Tea

Tea is second only to water as the most widely consumed beverage in the world. A great deal of attention has been directed to the polyphenolic constituents of tea, particularly green tea (Harbowy and Balentine, 1997). Polyphenols comprise up to 30 per cent of the total dry weight of fresh tea leaves. Catechins are the predominant and most significant of all tea polyphenols. The four major green tea catechins are epigallocatechin-3-gallate, epigallocatechin, epicatechin-3-gallate, and epicatechin.

Dreosti *et al.* (1997) stated that "no other agent tested for possible chemoprevention effects in animal models has elicited such strong activity as tea and its components at the concentrations usually consumed by humans."

There is some evidence that tea consumption may also reduce the risk of CVD. Tea consumption was the major source of flavonoids in a population of elderly men in the Netherlands. Intake of five flavonoids (quercetin, kaempferol, myricetin, apigenin, and luteolin), the majority of which was derived from tea consumption, was significantly inversely associated with mortality from CHD in this population. Although several other prospective studies have demonstrated a substantial reduction in CVD risk with tea consumption, the evidence is not presently conclusive.

## Functional Foods from Animal Sources

Although the vast number of naturally occurring health-enhancing substances are of plant origin, there are a number of physiologically-active components in animal products that deserve attention for their potential role in optimal health.

### Fish

Omega-3 (n-3) fatty acids are an essential class of polyunsaturated fatty acids (PUFAs) derived primarily from fish oil. The major PUFAs are eicosapentaenoic acid (EPA, C20:5, n3) and docosahexanoic acid (DHA, C22:6, n-3) (Prates and Mateus, 2002). DHA is an important part of the phospholipids of cellular membranes, especially in the brain and retina of the eye, and is essential for their functioning. DHA plays an important role in the development of brain and retina in infants. It has been suggested that the Western-type diet is currently deficient in n-3 fatty acids, which is reflected in the current estimated n-6 to n-3 dietary ratio of 20:25-1, compared to the 1:1 ratio on which humans evolved (Simopoulos, 1991). This has prompted researchers to examine the role of n-3 fatty acids in a number of diseases particularly cancer and CVD and more recently, in early human development.

The role of the omega-3 fatty acids in the human body are the followings:

1. Reduces the blood cholesterol and triglicerid levels
2. Reduces inflammation symptoms
3. Improves the efficiency of the immune system
4. Good effects on digestion
5. Reduces the risk of gastro- intestinal tumours, and helps cancer patients
6. Prevents premature birth
7. Better retina function
8. Reduces blood pressure
9. More effective digestion with increasing bile output
10. Reduces allergic diseases
11. Prevent diabetes

### Dairy Products

There is no doubt that dairy products are functional foods. They are one of the best sources of calcium, an essential nutrient which can prevent osteoporosis and possibly colon cancer. In view of the former, the National Academy of Sciences recently increased recommendations for this nutrient for most age groups. In addition to calcium, however, recent research has focused specifically on other components in dairy products, particularly fermented dairy products known as probiotics. Probiotics are defined as "live microbial feed supplements which beneficially affect the host animal by improving its intestinal microbial balance".

In addition to probiotics, there is growing interest in fermentable carbohydrates that feed the good microflora of the gut. The "nondigestible food ingredients that beneficially affect the host by selectively stimulating the growth and/or activity of one or a limited number of bacteria in the colon and thus improves host health," may include starches, dietary fibers, other non-absorbable sugars, sugar alcohols, and oligosaccharides. Of these, oligosaccharides have received the most attention, and numerous health benefits have been attributed to them. Oligosaccharides consist of short chain polysaccharides composed of three and 10 simple sugars linked together. They are found naturally in many fruits and vegetables (including banana, garlic, onions, milk, honey, artichokes). The prebiotic concept has been further extended to encompass the concept of synbiotic, a mixture of pro- and prebiotics. Many synbiotic products are currently on the market in Europion countries.

### Beef

An anticarcinogenic fatty acid known as conjugated linoleic acid (CLA) was first isolated from grilled beef in 1987. CLA refers to a mixture of positional and geometric isomers of linoleic acid (18:2 n-6) in which the double bonds are conjugated instead of existing in the typical methylene interrupted configuration. Nine different isomers of CLA have been reported as occurring naturally in food. CLA is unique in that it is found in highest concentrations in fat from ruminant animals (*e.g.*, beef, dairy, and lamb).

### Milk

It had made efforts to manipulate the CLA content of milk and animal tissue by changing the dietary composition. Such research can lead to the development of new high CLA containing functional foods'. Cows' milk fat is the richest common source of CLA.

### Designer Eggs

Eggs are of particular interest from a functionality point of view, because they are relatively rich in fatty acids and the associated fat-soluble compounds. The type and ratio of fatty acids is an important determinant of human health. The idea of egg enrichment with omega-3 fatty acids simultaneously with antioxidants and other vitamins has recently been used to produce VITA Eggs by Freshley Foods (Devon, UK).

## Conclusions

Increase in the evidence of supporting the observation that foods from animal origin containing physiologically active ingradients may enhance human health (Prates and Mateus, 2002). Diet is the most important component that have an impact on health. The field of functional foods is not well grown. Research into functional foods will advance in public health when the benefits of the functional foods are communicated to the consumer. The International Food Information

Council Foundation (Washington, D.C.) recently released a set of communication guidelines, aimed at scientists, journal editors, journalists, interest groups, and others for improving public understanding of emerging science. Finally, those foods whose health benefits are supported by sufficient scientific authentication have the potential to be an increasingly important component of a healthy lifestyle and to be beneficial to the public and the food industry.

## REFERENCES


Bellisle, F., Diplock, A. T., Hornstra, G., Koletzkos, B., Roberfroid, M., Salminen, S. and Saris, W.H.M. (1998). Functional food science in Europe. *British Journal of Nutrition,* **80**: S1-S193.

Block, G., Patterson, B. and Subar, A. (1992). Fruit, vegetables, and cancer prevention: A review of the epidemiological evidence. *Nutritional Cancer,* **18**; 1- 29.

Clinton, S.K. (1998). Lycopene: Chemistry, biology, and implications for human health and disease. Nutrition review, **56;** 35-51.

Clinton, S.K., Emenhiser, C., Schwartz, S.J., Bostwick, D.G., Williams, A.W., Moore, B.J. and Erdman, J.W. (1996). Cis-trans lycopene isomers, carotenoids, and retinol in the human prostate. Cancer Epidemiol. *Biomarkers Prev.* **5**; 823-833.

Clydesdale, F.M. (1997). A proposal for the establishment of scientific criteria for health claims for functional foods. *Nutrition Review,* **55** (12); 413-422 p.

Dreosti, *I.E.*, Wargovich, M.J., and Yang, C.S. 1997. Inhibition of carcinogenesis by tea: The evidence from experimental studies. *Critical Review Food Science Nutrition,* **37**;761- 770.

Elegbede, J.A., Maltzman, T.H., Elson, C.E. and Gould, M.N. (1993). Effects of anticarcinogenic monoterpenes on phase II hepatic metabolizing enzymes. *Carcinogenesis,* **14:** 1221-1223.

Giovannucci, E., Ascherio, A., Rimm, E.B., Stampfer, M.J., Colditz, G.A. and Willett, W.C. (1995). Intake of carotenoids and retinol in relation to risk of prostate cancer. *J. Natl. Cancer Inst,* **87**; 1767-1776.

Harbowy, M.E. and Balentine, D.A. (1997). Tea Chemistry. *Critical Review Plant Science,* **16**; 415-480.

Hasler, C.M. (2002). Functional foods: Benefits, concerns, challenges- A position paper from the American Council on Science and Health.

Nagourney, R.A. (1998). Garlic: Medicinal food or nutritious medicine? *Journal Medicinal Food,* **1**: 13-28.

Ofek, I., Goldhar, J., Zafriri, D., Lis, H., Adar, R. and Sharon, N. (1991). Anti- Escherichia coli adhesin activity of cranberry and blueberry juices. *New English Journal of Medicine,* **324;** 1599.

Prates, J.A.M. and Mateus, C.M.R.P. (2002). Functional foods from animal sources and their physiologically active components. *Revue Médical Véterinary*, **153**(3); 155-160 p.

Reuter H.D., Koch, H.P. and Lawson, L.D. (1996). Therapeutic effects and applications of garlic and its preparations. In: Garlic. The Science and Therapeutic Application of Allium sativum L. and Related Species, 2nd Ed., ed., H.P. Koch and L.D. Lawson, Williams and Wilkins, Baltimore.

Schmidt, D.R. and Sobota, A.E. (1988). An examination of the anti-adherence activity of cranberry juice on urinary and nonurinary bacterial isolates. *Microbios*. **55**; 173- 181.

Simopoulos, A.P. (1991). Omega-3 fatty acids in health and disease and in growth and development. *American Journal of Clinical Nutrition*, **54**; 438-463 p.

Steinmetz, K.A. and Potter, J.D. (1991). Vegetables, fruit, and cancer. II. Mechanisms. *Cancer Causes Control*, **2**(6); 427–442.

Thompson, L.U., Robb, P., Serraino, M. and Cheung, F. (1991). Mammalian lignan production from various foods. *Nutrition Cancer*, **16;** 43-52.

Tijburg, L.B.M., Mattern, T., Folts, J.D., Weisgerber, U.M., and Katan, M.B. (1997). Tea flavonoids and cardiovascular diseases: *A Critical Review Food Science Nutrition*, **37**; 771-785.

Verhoeven, D.T.H., Goldbohm, R.A., van Poppel, G., Verhagen, H. and van den Brandt, P.A. (1996). Epidemiological studies on brassica vegetables and cancer risk. *Cancer Epidemiology Biomarkers Prev*. **5**; 733-742.

Chapter 20

# Feeding Strategies to Enhance Milk Productivity in the Rural Areas

*R.P.S. Baghel, Sunil Nayak and Ankur Khare*

*Department of Animal Nutrition,
College of Veterinary Science and Animal Husbandry,
Nanaji Deshmukh Veterinary Science University, Jabalpur, Madhya Pradesh*

Milk is an important component of diets for all humans as it is high in essential amino acids that are most likely to be deficient in diets based on vegetable protein. Although milk is a high-cost source of protein and fat relative to vegetable sources, it is readily saleable particularly in the more affluent urban areas of developing countries. Improving milk production is therefore an important tool for improving the quality of life particularly for rural people in developing countries.

In spite of achieving the highest milk production (165.4 million tonnes in 2016-17) in the world, the performance of our cattle has been extremely poor. The country has a bovine population of 300 million as per 19th Livestock census 2012 and out of 190 million cattle population, 20 per cent are exotic and crossbreds (39 million) and about 80 per cent belonging to indigenous and Non-descript breeds. While India accounts for more than 18 per cent of the world population, the normal Indian cow with the poor farmer barely gives 1 to 2 litres per day. Thus 80 per cent of the cow population gives only 20 per cent of cow milk.

Milk production systems in our country are diverse. At the one extreme the systems are similar to those in most industrialized countries and are based on cows of high genetic potential given "high quality feeds" which include fodder crops/ silages and grain and protein concentrates. Milk production per cow is extremely high and technological inputs are high. At the other extreme are systems which are used by the vast majority of small farmers in India and are based on low inputs and productivity per cow is relatively low. These small-farmer systems vary from ones in which cows or buffaloes are fed on crop residues, agro-industrial by-products and roadside grass to beef cattle grazing tropical pastures that are milked once a day, with the calf having access to the dam for the other half of each day. In the latter systems, the pastures available to these `dual purpose' animals are typical of most tropical grasslands and are relatively low in protein and digestibility. A strategy for improving milk production in these systems has therefore two components. The first is to improve reproductive efficiency of the dairy animals and secondly to improve milk yield and persistency.

About 70 per cent of the milk producers in India are landless and marginal farmers and the disposable income from milk contributes significantly for sustaining their livelihood. A successful livestock production largely depends on continues supply of adequate, balanced and economic feeding. Feeding alone accounts for more than 70 per cent of the total cost of milk production; therefore, balanced feeding of dairy animals can play a pivotal role in successful livestock farming. To maximize profitability from the animals, one needs to ensure that these animals must receive the required quantity of protein, energy, minerals and vitamins, preferably from locally available feed resources.

Forage based economical feeding strategies are required to reduce the cost of quality livestock product as the feed alone constitutes 60-70 per cent of the milk production cost. Thus any attempt towards enhancing feed availability and economizing the feed cost would result in increased margin of profits to livestock owners also. There is tremendous pressure of livestock on available total feed and fodder, as land available for fodder production has been decreasing. At present, the country faces a net deficit of 35.6 per cent green fodder, 10.95 per cent dry crop residues and 44 per cent concentrate feed ingredients. To meet the current level of livestock production and its annual growth in population, the deficit in all components of fodder, dry crop residues and feed has to be met either from increasing productivity, utilizing untapped feed resources, increasing land area (may not possible due to human pressure for food crops) or through imports.

## Feed Resources Available to Livestock

Dairy animals in India and other tropical countries are fed mainly on by-products of various food crops, oil seeds and locally grown fodder. Due to population pressure the land for fodder production has dwindled alarmingly and the cereal crop residues like paddy straw, wheat straw, sorghum straw *etc.* have become the major source of feed for large sections of the ruminant population. The available resources are essentially low digestibility forages such as tropical pastures (both green and mature), straws and other crop residues and agricultural by-products which are generally low in protein. Fermentable energy and protein deficiencies in crop residues coupled with their low digestibility impair intake, ruminal functions, and thus animal productivity. The situation strongly demands the improvement of the nutritive value of high fibrous crop residues through various treatments, for the efficient utilization of existing feed resources.

## Management of Resources to Enhance Forage Productivity

Ample availability of feeds and fodders to livestock is vital for increasing the productivity. Feed is also the main input factor for milk and meat production form livestock constituting 60-70 per cent of the cost of livestock products. The inadequate feed resource is the major constraint in the productivity of livestock. Inadequate feed supply is coupled with the availability of low quality fibrous feed forming the major roughage source.

A large gap exists between demand and supply of feed and fodder in the country. At present, the country faces a net deficit of 35.6 per cent green fodder, 10.95 per cent dry crop residues and 44 per cent concentrate feed ingredients. Looking at the vast gap between the demand and supply position, it becomes necessary to put adequate efforts to transfer the potential technologies developed by various research organization in the country to farmer's field in order to increase the production and productivity of good quality fodder. To make dairying economically attractive, milk production and productivity has to be enhanced. This is possible only by making available good quality feed and fodder in adequate quantity. Fodder crops are the cheapest source of feed for livestock. Recently, through research efforts, a few feeding technologies have been developed with higher feed conversion efficiencies and having a potential for commercial manufacture, which can partially help in overcoming feed shortage in tropics and enhance animal productivity.

## Promoting Intensive Fodder Production

In India, the area under fodder cultivation has remained static for the last three decades at 4.5 per cent of the total cultivable land, due to pressure of human population. The only way to increase fodder production is through intensive fodder production, especially using high yielding varieties of fodder crops. Intercropping of cereal and a forage legume can serve the dual purpose of increased grain yield (wheat) and provide good grazing between harvest and ploughing, in place of unproductive fallow. Climbing pea planted with maize or sorghum not only increases that total quantity of Stover, but also improves its quality. The integration of forage crops in cropping system is the only way in the Indian context to increase green fodder supply for livestock. Integration of forage legumes improves soil fertility and soil structure and controls soil erosion and thus, helps in the sustainable development of agriculture (Reddy *et al.*, 2008).

## Top Feeds/Tree Leaves can act as Fodder Banks

Species of Leucaena, Glyceridia and Sespenia are excellent multipurpose rather wonder trees and bushes which can regularly provide high quality browse as well as serve as fodder bank. Their cultivation also improves soil fertility and the larger branches provide firewood. These trees can also be planted alongside roads and around ponds and edges of paddy fields, as well as in spaces not suitable for cultivation. Apart from these, many tropical trees like prosopis juliflora and Acacia nilotica could be raised on saline soils with gypsum and farmyard manure and serve as green forage (top feed) for the livestock.

## Encouraging Silvipastoral System and Grassland Development

Although the land base for livestock has been shrinking in Indian, which can be attributed to various kinds of pressures, the possibility still exists to obtain more herbage from about 60 m ha of the country's land area, through silvi-pasture system and better grassland management. An integrated system of agro-forestry system in which legumes, pulses (pigeon pea) and grasses can be show in association with fodder tree like *Leucaena leucocephala*, can provide fodder without any reduction in pulses yield. Similarly, Guinea grass could successfully be grown under coconut plantation, or pasture grass like stylo or citrus or cowpea can be cultivated in the first few years of plantation of citrus or zizyphus (Reddy *et al.*, 2008). Improvement of degraded grasslands and rehabilitation of problematic soils like saline, acidic and heavy soils through vegetative cover should be the priority of the planners. Apart from improving the fertility status of the soil by introducing suitable legumes, grasslands require regeneration through the process of natural recovery by closure/exclusion of biotic interference. This would involve fencing of the area, establishment of soil and moisture conservation structures to support natural regeneration such as contour bonding, furrowing, ploughing, fertilization *etc.* This can also help in minimizing erosion of these lands and produce biomass which shall be much cheaper to support animal production.

## Exploiting the Genetic Variability in Nutritional Quality of Straws

A large variation in straw quality exists among cultivars with respect to in vitro and in situ DM digestibility (Capper, 1988). This variation could be as high as 10-15 units, which has been studied in most of the cereal crop residues *viz.* rice, wheat, barley, sorghum and millets. In the crop-livestock sustainable production system, better quality of straw can result in 10 per cent increase in productivity of ruminants. Cereal breeders have often overlooked this point. It is high time that the cereal breeders plan their breeding programs in collaboration with animal nutritionists, and thus, help in improving the economic lot of resource poor farmers.

## Nutritional Evaluation of Forage Resources and Development of Feeding Strategies

Poor quality crop residues are still major source of livestock feed, leaving animals undernourished, which increase their susceptibility to diseases, lowering reproduction efficiency ultimately affecting milk, and meat production for human beings, which is a matter of great concern for the country. It is concerned to develop forage based feeding systems for optimum and efficient productive and reproductive performances in different categories of livestock, development of technology for efficient conservation of surplus green grass/biomass available during rainy season, rumen manipulation and improvement of low grade forages/ roughages for improved livestock production and nutrient (protein and energy) management and monitoring blood minerals status in milch animals fed low grade forages.

## Improving Nutritive Value of Crop Residue by Urea Treatment

Crop residues (wheat straw, rice straw, stovers, *etc.*) characterized by high indigestible fibre due to increased lignification of cellulose. Fermentable energy and protein deficiencies in crop residues coupled with their low digestibility impair intake, ruminal functions, and thus animal productivity. The situation strongly demands the improvement of the nutritive value of high fibrous crop residues through various treatments, for the efficient utilization of existing feed resources. Out of the several chemicals tried for cleaving the lingo-cellulosic bonds in fibrous crop residues and improve their digestibility, urea/ammonia treatment has emerged as the most effective one and is particularly more feasible under tropical situation. Urea, when used for treatment of straw enhances the nutritional quality of straw in terms of increased nitrogen content, improved palatability and digestibility of straw (Sharma *et al.,* 2004).

## Use of Urea Molasses Mineral Block Licks (UMMB)

Urea molasses mineral block is prepared by mixing urea, molasses, mineral mixture and other ingredients in a suitable proportion. It is a readily available source of energy, protein and minerals for the dairy animal. Supplementing an animal with UMMB would provide adequate quantity of these nutrients and slow ingestion of urea leads to efficient microbial protein production and improved digestibility.

## Use of Densified Complete Feed Block

Concept of densified complete feeds with fibrous crop residues is a noble way to incr ease the intake and improves th e nutrients utilization. A complete feed block has been defined as a system of feeding all ingredients including roughages, processed and mixed uniformly, to be made available *ad lib* to the animals. The feeding of complete feed stabilizes rumen fermentation, minimizes fermentation loss and ensures better ammonia utilization (Prasad *et al.,* 2001). This pattern of rumen fermentation enhances utilization of poor quality roughage and improves the palatability of unconventional feeds.

This is an innovative food technology, rather a novel nutrient delivery system by which animal can get all the required nutrients for 24 hours as a balanced ration. The dry roughage and the concentrate are the two major components and the micronutrient supplements form the third, minor component. The technology allows all the ingredients (major or minor) to get sufficiently blended so that the concentrate particulate matter sticks to fibre particles with the help of binder or molasses. This helps in preventing the separation of ingredients, making it as much as a homogenous feed and leaving little scope for the selectivity by the animal. The combined feed is enriched (value added) with necessary mineral and vitamin supplements and feed additives, making it a wholesome complete balanced ration for a specific category of dairy stock. This technology is very much helpful in areas that face an acute shortage of feed or fodder particularly during natural calamities like draught and flood situations.

## Feeding of Bypass Nutrients (Protein and Fat)

Dairy animals have four compartments in its stomach. The first and the foremost is 'rumen' where most of the feed items are degraded. Around 60 to 70 per cent of dietary protein meals fed to animals are degraded to ammonia in the rumen. A significant part of this ammonia is excreted through urine in the form of urea. Thus, a large portion of protein from expensive cakes/meals is wasted. If suitable treatment is given to dietary protein meals, degradation in the rumen can be minimised. This process or treatment to protect dietary protein from degradation in rumen is known as bypass protein technology. These protected meals are digested more efficiently in the small intestine and results in extra protein being available for milk production. This helps the animal to produce more milk and of optimum quality.

When the technology of bypass nutrients was introduced and successfully applied in Australia and other western countries, about three decades back, it was thought that the technologies are suitable for only high yielding animals. Even the western experts advised us against the use of bypass protein in Indian, in view of the low production potential of our animals, and enough microbial protein being synthesized in rumen.

With regard to bypass protein, more than two decades of research work, involving number of trials conducted on medium producing cattle, buffalo, goats for growth, milk production, feed efficiency reproductive efficiency, animal health, milk composition and milk quality all have established that feeding of bypass protein is very much relevant to Indian/tropical situation (Walli, 2008). What the western experts over looked was the fact that more than the shortage of amino acids, energy is the limiting factor in the optimum production of our ruminant stock. Very high levels of ruminal ammonia invariably found in Indian ruminant stock than the optimum required level of 5mg/100 ml rumen liquor, provided the key that there is not sufficient energy available in rumen to trap this ammonia into bacterial protein. Feeding of bypass protein not only saves dietary proteins form excessive degradation to ammonia, most of which is lost as urea through urine, but supplies more amino acids to the animal. The extra amino acids are converted to glucose in liver to compensate for the inadequate energy supply to dairy animals in tropical countries, and thereby boost up their production. By pass protein thus, has emerged as the cheapest feeding technology for feeding ruminants, especially the dairy animals, which is now a successful commercial feed technology in India, pushing up the milk yield by 10-15 per cent (Walli, 2008).

As far the bypass fat technology, the indigenous production is still lacking and the country is depending on imports. May be technology can be made cost effective if cheaper oil sources are used. Again, earlier it was thought that this technology is suitable only for high yielding animals, but that notion has been proved wrong through the number of trials conducted on medium producing cows and buffalos fed bypass fat supplements. The bypass fat supplies concentrated form of energy and thus, compensates for the inadequate supply of energy form the original diet. The sufficient energy supply boosts up milk production in energy limiting animals. The increase in milk yield is from 10-25 per cent (Thakur and Shelke, 2010).

Apart from significant increase in milk production, feeding of bypass fat has several added advantages to the farmer. The animal exhibits regularity in reproductive cycle, reducing the inter-calving period to the desired minimum. During the summer months, feeding of bypass fat also helps the animal to fight heat stress because when bypass fat is fed to the animal the amount of straw consumption goes down, which otherwise produces excessive heat of fermentation in rumen and animal starts panting. Through several feeding trials, it has become clear that feeding of bypass fat even to medium producing animals receiving with the additional advantage of increasing the reproductive efficiency and more importantly, guarding the animal against heat stress.

## Encouraging the Use of Area Specific Mineral Mixture

Minerals are required by dairy animals for their metabolic functions, growth, milk production, reproduction and health. Animal cannot synthesize minerals inside its body and majority of the feeds generally available in India and other tropical countries are deficient in mineral content, especially trace minerals. Also, the intensive crop production for the last four decades has caused an imbalance of minerals in the soils, which not only affect the growth of plants, but causes mineral deficiency in animals as well. The lower intake of mineral by the animals can lead to their suboptimal growth, production and reproduction.

Surveys conducted recently in different regions of India have clearly brought out two things to the fore. Firstly, that the mineral deficiencies very form region to region and secondly, that the dairy farmers in Indian, by and large, are not aware of the importance of feeding mineral mixture to their animals (Gowda *et al.*, 2008). The dairy animals in the rural areas invariably have the problem of repeat breeding, which can be mostly attributed to mineral deficiencies, especially that of trace minerals. On-farm trials conducted by various research groups in the rural areas on minerals supplementation to animals have yielded positive results in term of improvements in reproductive efficiency of these animals and also in their better productive performance. The deficiency of minerals/trace minerals varies from region to region in the country. Level of minerals in feeds and fodder varies from region to region, thus mineral availability to the animal also varies. So, it is necessary to produce region specific mineral mixture accordingly. Therefore, animal should be supplemented with adequate amount of good quality mineral mixture in their ration. We need to develop region specific mineral/trace minerals supplements, based on the survey conducted in each region. The trace minerals are now available in chealated from. In this form, these trace minerals like Zn, Cu, Mn and Co are more effective, having better absorbability and improved bio-availability. There is an urgent need for the extension agencies in the country to educate the farmers about the benefits of feeding mineral mixture/chealated minerals to their livestock, so that their livestock can perform at optimum level with respect to production as well as reproduction.

## Recommending Selective Use of Feed Additives

Several feed additives (supplements) have been developed for livestock, and some of these are now commercially available in the market. These supplements appear to be promising, but more research trials are required to be conducted at the research centers to see their suitability as well as economic feasibility under field conditions. Probiotic live yeast cultures are especially effective in enhancing fibre digestion in a situation, where high concentrate feeding is pursued. The technology is more likely to be useful for animals getting low-fibre high-concentrate diets, whereas in the tropical countries, the majority of resource poor farmers are using straw based diets for feeding of bovine stock. Though it may still be useful at large farms, where, due to insufficiency of green fodder, high concentrates feeding is followed. However, probiotic rumen anaerobic fungi appear to be very promising, because of the higher activity of the polysaccharide degrading enzymes, they possess. At present, the efforts are on to exploit this technology for commercial purpose, using the spores of the fungi in the feed rather that the organism as such, because of longer shelf life of the spores (Sehgal and Jha, 2008). This technology requires further microbiological research to make the spores commercially available in the market. Commercially produced fibrolytic enzymes, like cellulose and xylanase, are now available in the market at a cheaper price. The enzyme supplementation significantly increases the growth rate of calves and the performance of lactating animals. Recently, some non-ionic surfactants (NIS) have also been reported to increase the productivity of dairy animals, in terms of both growth rate and milk production, through the relèase of more fibre degrading enzymes from bacterial cell in rumen, resulting in more fibre digestion.

## Reducing Methane Emission through Dietary Interventions

The conditions under which the high density ruminant stock is reared in India and other tropical countries, are conducive for release of high levels of methane from enteric/rumen fermentation into the atmosphere. It calls for making efforts to reduce these levels of emission through technical intervention such as supplementation, fibre fortications and fibre polarization (Padmakumar, 2008). Lately, some herbal extracts, including the supplements containing spices like fenugreek seeds and garlic extracts have been shown to have some positive effect on rumen metabolism, including the defaunation and ruminal methane reduction (Bhatta *et al.,* 2013). The advantage of feeding a balanced ration having a good proportion of concentrate with straw, as in feed block also results in less methane production in rumen. Newer technologies like straw based densified complete feed block, which provides a balanced ration or the feeding of bypass nutrients like bypass protein and bypass fat, do help in reducing methane emission. The letter two technologies also help animals to fight heat stress during hot and hot humid conditions.

## Conclusion

In the tropical countries, feed shortage, especially the shortage of quality feeds is a serious problem. For increasing the supply of green herbage, the strategies needed are: conservation of degraded pasturelands and development of wastelands, even introducing shrubs and trees, to provide top feeds for livestock. Feeding strategies for ruminants in tropics should also include environmental protection, through reduced methane emission, apart from increasing the productivity of ruminant stock. Some feeding technologies are commercially available today, *viz.* feeding of bypass nutrients and densified TMR, which can boost up the productivity of ruminant stock and also reduce methane emission.

## REFERENCES

Bhatta, R., Saravanan, M., Baruah, L., Sampath, K.T., and Prasad C.S. (2013). Effect of plant secondary compounds on in vitro methane, ammonia production and ruminal protozoa population. *J Appl Microbiol.,* 115(2): 455-65.

Capper, B.S. (1988). Genetic variation in the feeding value of cereal straw. *Anim. Feed Sci. Technol.* 21: 127-140.

Gowda, N.K.S., Prasad, C.S., Selvaraju, S., Reddy, I.J., Ananthram, K. and Sampath, K.T. (2008). Feeding practices and nutrient status of dairy cows in adopted villages under institute village linkage programme. *Indian Vet. J.,* 85: 745-748.

Padmakumar,V. (2008). Livestock, livelihood and environment: The policy context and challenges. XXXVI Dairy Industry Conference, BHU, pp. 50-56.

Prasad, C. S., Gowda, N. K. S. and Rammana, J.V. (2001). Feeding strategies to enhance animal productivity. In; *Proceedings of the 10th Animal Nutrition Conference, NDRI, Karnal, India*, pp. 23-45.

Reddy, D. V., Elanchezhian, (2008). Evaluation of tropical tree leaves as ruminant feedstuff based on cell contents, cell wall fractions and polyphenolic compounds. *Livest. Res. Rural Dev.,* 20 (5): 77

Sharma, K., Dutta, N. and Naulia, U. (2004). An on-farm appraisal of feeding urea-treated straw to buffaloes during late pregnancy and lactation in a mixed farming system. *Livest. Res. Rural Dev.* 16(11).

Thakur, S.S. and Shelke, S.K. (2010). Effect of supplementing bypass fat prepared from soybean acid oil on milk yield and nutrient utilization in Murrah buffaloes. *Indian J. Anim. Sci.,* 80 (4): 354-357.

Walli, T.K. (2008). Densified TMR – A newer nutrient delivery system for feeding dairy animals in tropics. In *Proc. XXXVI Dairy Industry Conference*, pp. 74–79. BHU, Varanasi, India.

## Chapter 21

# Hydroponics: An Alternative to Cultivated Green Fodder

*Sunil Nayak, R.P.S. Baghel and Ankur Khare*

*Department of Animal Nutrition*
*College of Veterinary Science and Animal Husbandry,*
*Nanaji Deshmukh Veterinary Science University, Jabalpur, Madhya Pradesh*

## Introduction

In India, livestock plays an important role for the nutritional security, particularly of the small and marginal farmers. Increase in the livestock population along with the intensive rearing system has resulted in the increase demands for feeds and fodder in the country. The feed scarcity has been the main limiting factor in improving the livestock productivity (Brithal and Jha, 2005). The land allocation for cultivation of green fodder is limited to only 5 per cent of the gross cropped area; but by 2020, India would require a total 526, 855 and 56 million tons of dry matter, green fodder and concentrates (Dikshit and Brithal, 2010).

The productive and reproductive efficiency of the livestock is adversely affected due to the unavailability of good quality green fodder. Besides the unavailability of land, more labour requirement for cultivation (sowing, earthing up, weeding, harvesting *etc.*), more growth time, non-availability of same quality round the year, requirement of manure and fertilizer; the uncertain rain fall, water scarcity and natural calamities due to climate change are the major constraints for green fodder production by the livestock farmers. Due to the above constraints of the conventional method of fodder cultivation, hydroponics technology is coming up as an alternative to grow fodder for farm animals (Naik *et al.,* 2011; Naik, 2012;

Naik *et al.,* 2013). Further, hydroponics technology for fodder production will be very effective for rearing small ruminants (sheep and goats) as these animals have lesser dry matter requirement and are being shifted from extensive to intensive rearing system.

Hydroponic fodder is essentially the germination of a seed (such as malt barley or oats) and sprouted into a high quality, highly nutritious, disease free animal food. This process takes place in a very versatile and intensive hydroponic growing unit where only water and nutrients are used to produce a grass and root combination that is very lush and high in nutrients. This green fodder is extremely high in protein and metabolisable energy, which is highly digestible by most animals. The word hydroponics has been derived from the Greek word 'water working'. Hydro means 'water' and ponic means 'working' and it is a technology of sprouting grains or growing plants without soil, but only with water or nutrient rich solution.

Fodder crops produced by hydroponics technology are also known as hydroponics fodder, sprouted fodder or sprouted grain. Sprouting of the grains is made inside a greenhouse within a short period of approximately seven days. A greenhouse is a framed or inflated structure covered with a transparent or translucent material in which the crops could be grown under the conditions at least partially controlled environment and which is large enough to permit a person to work within it to carry out cultural operations (Chandra and Gupta, 2003).

## Fodder Crops used for Hydroponics

Different types of fodder crops *viz.* barley (Reddy *et al.,* 1988), oats, wheat (Snow *et al.,* 2008); sorghum, alfalfa, cowpea (Al-Karaki and Al-Hashimi, 2012) and maize (Naik *et al.,* 2011; Naik *et al.,* 2012a) can be produced by hydroponics technology. However, the choice of the hydroponics fodder to be produced depends on the geographical and agro-climatic conditions and easy availability of seeds. In India, maize grain should be the choice as the grain for production of hydroponics fodder due to its easy availability, lower cost, good biomass production and quick growing habit. The grain should be clean, sound, undamaged or free from insect infestation, untreated, viable and of good quality for better biomass production.

## Seed Preparation

Soaking of seeds and the rapid uptake of water for facilitating the metabolism and utilization of reserve materials of the seeds for growth and development of the plants is a very important step for production of hydroponics forage. In case of barley (Morgan *et al.,*1992) and maize (Naik, 2012b) seeds, 4 hours soaking in water is beneficial. Under field conditions, farmers producing hydroponics maize forage have the practice of putting the seeds in a gunny bag tightly and then make it wet and keep for 1-2 days.

## Seed Rate

The seed rate also affects the yield of the hydroponics fodder which varies with the type of seeds. Most of the commercial units recommend seed rate of 6-8 kg/m2 (Morgan *et al.*, 1992), however, seed rate of 7.6 kg/m2 has been suggested by Naik (2012) for hydroponics maize fodder for higher output. If seed density is high, there are more chances of microbial contamination in the root mat which affects the growth of the sprouts.

## Production of Hydroponics Fodder

### Principle

Hydroponic fodder production involves supplying cereal grain with necessary moisture and nutrients, to enable germination and plant growth in the absence of a solid growing medium. The resulting green shoots and root mat are harvested and fed to livestock. The grain responds to the supply of moisture and nutrients by germinating, sprouting and then producing a 200 – 250mm long vegetative green shoot with interwoven roots within 5 to 8 days. A range of cereals can be utilized for fodder production, including barley, oats, wheat and maize. The most commonly used cereal grain is barley. Barley fodder systems are the focus of the analysis within this report. There are a range of chemical and structural changes that take place within the cereal grain through the hydroponic growing process. Activation of enzymes within the grain leads to hydrolysis of proteins, carbohydrates and lipids into their simpler components (Dung, Godwin, and Nolan, 2010). This hydrolysis increases the concentrations of amino acids, soluble sugars and fatty acids within the grain and resulting shoot (Chavan and Kadam, 1989). The amount of sprouts produced (yield) and quality of the fodder is influenced by a number of factors including:

1. Grain - grain quality, grain variety and treatments
2. Growing environment - temperature, humidity and incidence of mould
3. Management of the system - water quality and pH, soaking time, nutrient supply, depth and density of grain in troughs, and growing duration (Sneath and McIntosh, 2003).

### Production Systems

Hydroponics is produced in greenhouses under controlled environment within a short period (Sneath and McIntosh, 2003). A greenhouse is a framed or inflated structure covered with a transparent or translucent material in which the crops could be grown under the conditions of at least partially controlled environment. However, the structure should be large enough to permit a person to carry out cultural operations (Chandra and Gupta, 2003). The greenhouse for the production of hydroponics fodder can be of hi-tech greenhouse type or low cost greenhouse type as per the financial status of the farmer and availability of building material.

#### (i) Hi-tech greenhouse type hydroponics fodder cultivation unit

The hi-tech greenhouse type unit consists of a control unit and may be used with or without air conditioner. The control unit regulates input of water and light automatically through sensors. Although all types of fodder crops can be grown in the hi-tech green house but the routine operational cost is more particularly for sprouting the *rabi* crops (barley, oat, wheat *etc.*). This is because of the requirement for air conditioner in the hydroponics system to maintain cold and dry environment.

**(ii) Low cost greenhouse type hydroponics fodder cultivation unit**

Hydroponics fodder can also be produced in low cost greenhouses or devices (Naik *et al.,* 2013c). The low cost greenhouses or shade net structures can be prepared from bamboo, wood, MS steel or galvanized iron steel. The cost of the shade net structures depends upon the type of fabricating material but is significantly lower than the hi-tech greenhouses.

The daily operation of the fodder shed revolves around 6 main tasks:

**i. Harvesting mature fodder**

Mature fodder is pulled out of the trays as a complete mat. It is commonly loaded on a cart and wheeled out the end of the fodder shed and loaded onto a vehicle or trailer for feeding.

**ii. Cleaning Trays**

It is critical that the trays and all equipment are thoroughly cleaned to reduce the risk of mould and other infections. A water blaster is commonly used to achieve this.

**iii. Sowing new grain**

New grain, which has been soaked for 24 hours, is sown into the trays. This grain is sown in an even layer 3cm deep.

**iv. Adjusting nutrient flows**

Nutrient flows are adjusted across each stack. The water and nutrient requirements of the growing fodder increases each day and thus the flow to each tray must be adjusted to ensure appropriate water and nutrient supply for the growing fodder. Small taps into each tray are adjusted to achieve this.

**v. Topping up nutrient and acid supplies**

Nutrient is added to the nutrient tank via an automated system. The pH of the nutrient solution is also maintained via an automated system. Thus, there is a need to check that the supply of nutrient concentrate and acid is adequate to supply the systems needs.

**vi. Feeding out**

The fodder is fed out to the appropriate stock class. This is commonly fed out in its mat form. A farmer in the Mackenzie Basin has trialed mulching the fodder first to improve utilization by the sheep but observed no real advantage in utilization. The labour requirements for fodder sheds depend largely on the level of automation

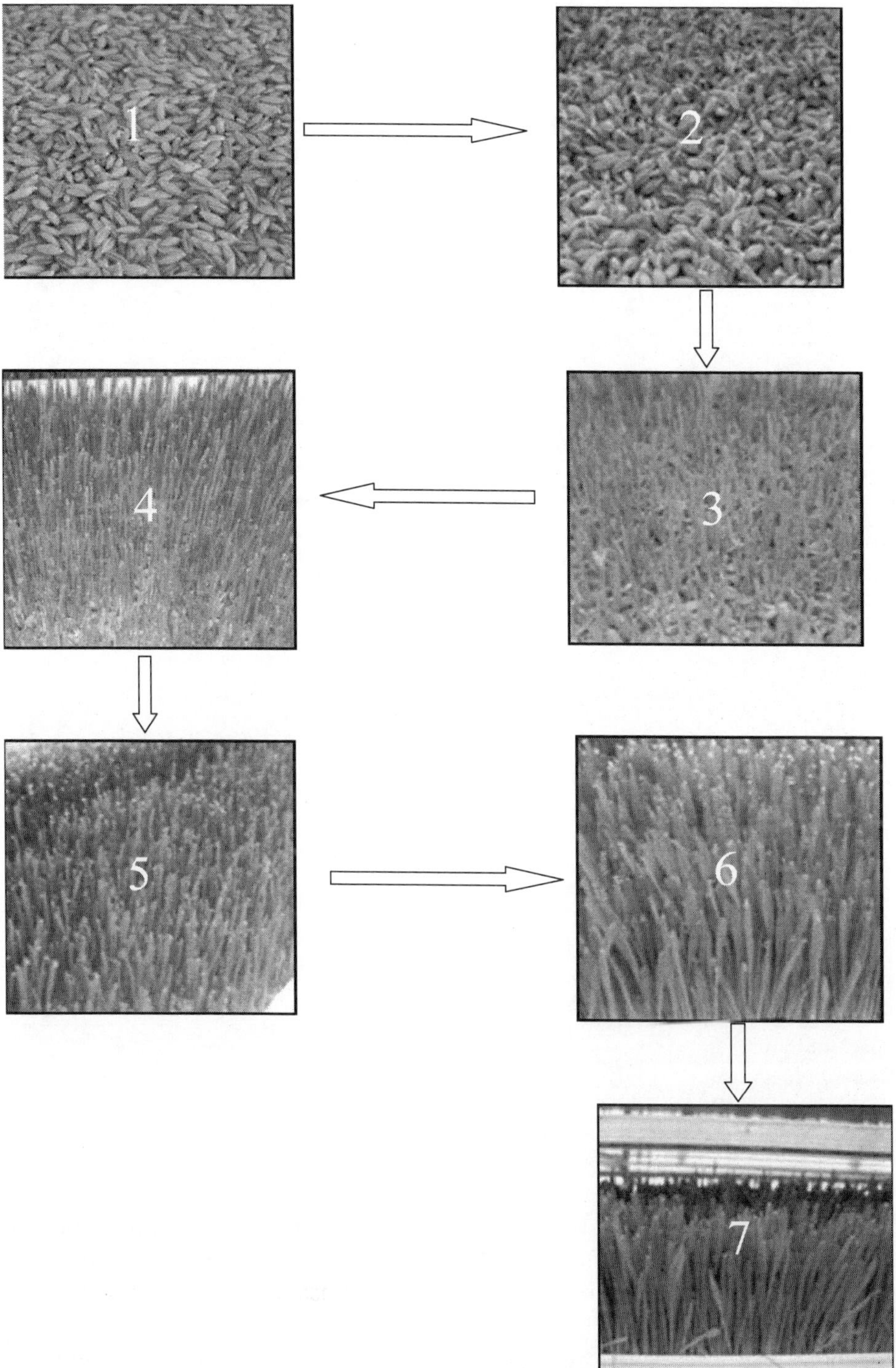


**Figure 21.1. Change of Grain at 1 Day to Green Leafy Hydroponics Fodder at 7 Day.**

within the system. The suggested daily labour requirement to operate a mid-sized system, producing 1 ton of wet feed per day and based on the set up and operation outlined above varies from 2 to 4 hours per day (Sneath and McIntosh, 2003).

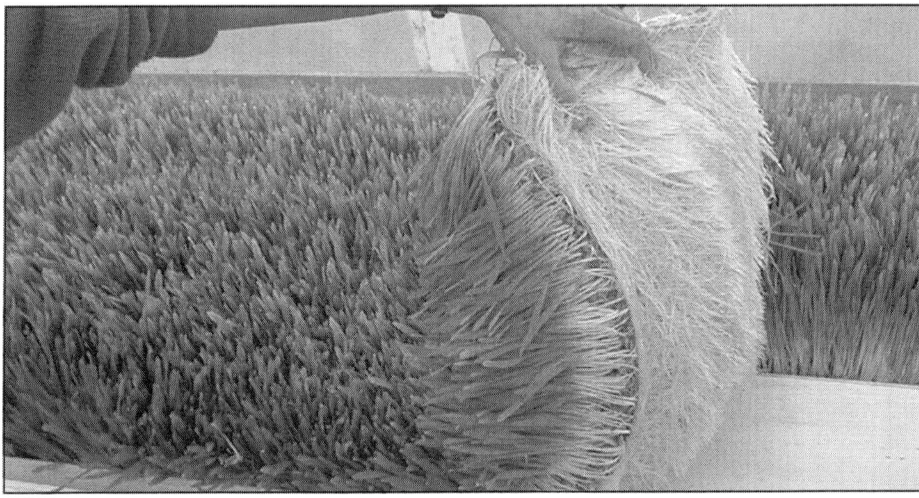

**Figure 21.2. Barley Fodder Harvested as a Single Mat.**

## Hydroponic Fodder Nutritional Attribute Analysis

To compare the relative economic viability of fodder it is necessary to consider its nutritional attributes to analyze its value as a feed source for livestock. The Table 21.1 presents nutrient analyses for a range of feed types, including hydroponic fodder:

**Table 21.1. Nutrient Content of a Range of Feed Sources**

| *Feed* | *Dry Matter (per cent)* | *Metabolisable Energy (MJME/kg DM)* | *Crude Protein (CP per cent)* |
|---|---|---|---|
| Barley Grain | 88 | 12 | 10 |
| Barley Straw | 89 | 6 | 2 |
| Pasture Silage | 43 | 9 | 14 |
| Pasture Hay | 86 | 8 | 10 |
| Barley Fodder | 9.9 | 11 | 24 |

The changes in the nutrient content during the growth of hydroponics fodder maize have been given in Table 21.2. Observations clearly indicate increase in nutritive value of hydroponics fodder maize as compared to conventional maize fodder.

**Table 21.2. Nutrient Content (per cent DM basis) of Hydroponics Maize Fodder**

| *Nutrient* | *Maize Seed (0 day)* | *Days of Sprouting under Hydroponics System* | | | | | | | *Conventional Maize Fodder* |
|---|---|---|---|---|---|---|---|---|---|
| | | *1* | *2* | *3* | *4* | *5* | *6* | *7* | |
| CP | $8.60^{a}$ | $8.88^{a}$ | $9.14^{ab}$ | $9.65^{b}$ | $11.27^{d}$ | $11.58^{d}$ | $12.89^{e}$ | $13.57^{f}$ | $10.67^{c}$ |
| **EE** | $2.56^{abc}$ | $2.49^{ab}$ | $2.57^{abc}$ | $2.88^{bcd}$ | $3.08^{cde}$ | $3.06^{cde}$ | $3.21^{e}$ | $3.49^{e}$ | $2.27^{a}$ |
| **CF** | $2.50^{a}$ | $2.55^{a}$ | $3.07^{a}$ | $4.72^{b}$ | $5.51^{c}$ | $7.56^{d}$ | $10.67^{c}$ | $14.07^{f}$ | $25.92^{g}$ |
| **NFE** | $84.49^{b}$ | $84.15^{h}$ | $82.87^{g}$ | $79.20^{f}$ | $77.65^{c}$ | $74.04^{d}$ | $69.21^{c}$ | $66.72^{b}$ | $51.78^{a}$ |
| **TA** | $1.57^{a}$ | $1.67^{a}$ | $1.84^{ab}$ | $1.92^{ab}$ | $2.19^{bc}$ | $2.44^{c}$ | $3.34^{d}$ | $3.84^{d}$ | $9.36^{f}$ |
| **AIA** | $0.02^{a}$ | $0.03^{a}$ | $0.08^{a}$ | $0.09^{a}$ | $0.13^{a}$ | $0.14^{a}$ | $0.24^{a}$ | $0.33^{a}$ | $1.40^{b}$ |

***a,b,c,d,e,f**: Means bearing different superscripts in the same row differ significantly ($p<0.05$).

## Yield

There are a wide range of claims regarding to the productive yield of hydroponic fodder systems. These range from 6 to 10 times the weight of green fodder harvested relative to the weight of grain sown (Sneath and McIntosh, 2003). The wet yield, while interesting, does not provide an accurate measure of the feed value of the fodder. To get an accurate understanding, there is a need to calculate the dry matter yield. The yield, on a Dry Matter (DM) basis, is dependent on the weight of sprouts grown from a given weight of grain and the DM per cent of the sprouts (Sneath and McIntosh, 2003).

An analysis completed on hydroponic fodder from a shed operated in the MacKenzie Basin showed a dry matter content of 9.9 per cent. This means that for every tonne of fodder produced, there is 99 kg of dry matter. Assuming a generous yield of eight times the weight of grain, this 1 tonne of green fodder would require 125 kg of barley grain. Assuming the grain is 90 per cent DM, this equates to an input of 112.5 kg DM, for an output of 99 kg DM. This is a loss of 12 per cent of original DM weight and supports the findings of previous research. Dung *et al.* (2010) reported that there is no record of any cases where the DM yield of the sprouts was higher than that of the original grain.

## Digestibility

A study in 1992 measured the digestibility of barley grain and sprouts at differing ages. The results of this are presented below (Table 21.3), and suggest that, other than at 4 days old, there is no real advantage in sprouting barley to improve digestibility.

**Table 21.3. The Digestibility of Barley Sprouts of differing Age**

| | *Organic Matter* | *Dry Matter* | *In vivo* |
|---|---|---|---|
| Grain | 88.8 per cent | 89.9 per cent | 83.9 per cent |
| 4 days | 91.8 per cent | 92.2 per cent | 85.8 per cent |
| 6 days | 87.9 per cent | 88.9 per cent | 82.1 per cent |
| 8 days | 88.4 per cent | 89.0 per cent | 82.6 per cent |

## Energy

Processed grain (cracked) and sprouts are both highly digestible and nutritious feeds. The process of sprouting the grain turns the starch in the grain to sugars in the sprouts (Sneath and McIntosh, 2003). Work by Dung *et al.* (2010) found that the energy value of the sprouts was also lower than that of the grain on a DM basis, with a gross energy loss of 2 per cent recorded after comparing the sprouts with the original grain.

## Protein

Protein is a critical element for animal growth and performance and is very important in analyzing the feed value of fodder. The effect of sprouting on protein content isn't clear, with some studies illustrating increases in protein, and others decreases in protein. In one of the latest fodder studies, Dung *et al.* (2010) found crude protein, ash and all other minerals except potassium were higher in concentration on a DM basis in the sprouts than in the barley grain (Dung *et al.*, 2010). This illustrates an advantage to the fodder.

**Table 21.4. Dry Matter, Ash and Crude Protein Contents of Seed and 4, 6 and 8-day Old Barley Grass Mats**

| | *Dry Matter (per cent of input)* | *Ash (g/kg DM)* | *Crude Protein (per cent DM)* |
|---|---|---|---|
| Original Seed | 100 | 21 | 10.1 |
| 4 Day Old Fodder | 96 | 22 | 10.8 |
| 6 Day Old Fodder | 91 | 31 | 13.7 |
| 8 Day Old Fodder | 84 | 53 | 14.9 |

## Vitamins

The vitamin content is generally improved by sprouting. This may make little difference to the feed value though, with Sneath and McIntosh (2003), reporting that the increases in individual vitamins are so small that its practical significance in meeting the nutritional requirements of cereal-based diets is difficult to evaluate in feeding trials. The Table 21.5 displays the quantitative changes in vitamin content of barley grain and 6 day old fodder. It is clearly evident that there is a significant increase in Vitamin content, but the value of that increase is not clear.

**Table 21.5. Vitamin Analysis of Grain and 6 Day Old Fodder**

| | *Grain* | *Barley Fodder* |
|---|---|---|
| Vitamin E | 7.40 | 62.4 |
| Beta – carotene | 4.10 | 42.7 |
| Biotin | 0.16 | 1.15 |
| Free Folic Acid | 0.12 | 1.05 |

## Animal Performance on Hydroponic Fodder

A wide range of trials to assess livestock performance on spouts have been conducted globally. These have included the performance of dairy cattle, beef cattle, pigs and poultry (Sneath and McIntosh, 2003). In their comprehensive review of hydroponic fodder in relation to beef cattle, Sneath and McIntosh (2003) reported that most of the trials on livestock performance from hydroponic sprouts show no advantage to including them in the diet, especially when it replaces highly nutritious feeds such as grain.

Observations in Table 21.6 indicate that feeding of hydroponics fodder increased the digestibility of the nutrients of the ration which could be attributed to the tenderness of the fodder (Reddy *et al.*, 1988; Naik *et al.*, 2014). The digestibility of the nutrients of the hydroponics fodder was comparable with the highly digestible legumes like berseem and other clovers (Pandey and Pathak, 1991). The DCP and TDN contents of the hydroponics barley fodder were optimum to meet the production requirement of the lactating cows (Reddy *et al.*, 1988).

**Table 21.6. Effect of Feeding of Hydroponics Fodder on Intake and Digestibility of Nutrients**

| *Parameter* | *Hydroponics Fodder* | | *Reference* |
|---|---|---|---|
| | *No* | *Yes* | |
| **Digestibility (per cent)** | | | |
| DM | 60.34-61.15 | 64.48-65.53 | Reddy *et al.* (1988)<br>Pandey and Pathak (1991)<br>Fazaeli *et al.* (2011)<br>Naik *et al.* (2014) |
| OM | 61.89-64.19 | 65.98-68.47 | |
| CP | 61.89-68.86 | 66.77-72.46 | |
| EE | 69.92-82.05 | 77.60-87.69 | |
| CF | 47.93-53.25 | 54.85-59.21 | |
| NFE | 65.84-67.37 | 68.13-70.47 | |
| **Nutritive Value (per cent)** | | | |
| DCP | 6.89-8.61 | 7.82-9.65 | |
| TDN | 55.43-64.00 | 61.19-73.12 | |
| NR | - | 6.72 | |
| **Nutrient Intake (kg/d)** | | | |
| CP | - | 0.97 | |
| DCP | - | 0.67 | |
| TDN | - | 5.20 | |

The hydroponics fodders have good palatability. The germinated seeds embedded in the root system are also consumed along with the shoots of the plants, so there is no nutrient wasting. The intake of fresh hydroponics maize fodder by dairy cows may be up to 25 kg/animal/day along with limited concentrate mixture and sorghum straw. Supplementation of the hydroponics fodder in the ration of the dairy cows improves digestibility of nutrients and milk yield in dairy cows (Table 21.7).

**Table 21.7. Effect of Supplementation of Hydroponics Naize Fodder on Digestibility of Nutrients and Milk Yield of Dairy Cows**

| *Parameters* | *Hydroponics Fodder* | | *per cent increase* |
|---|---|---|---|
| | - | + | |
| **Digestibility (per cent)** | | | |
| Dry matter | 61.15 | 65.39 | 6.94 |
| Organic matter | 64.19 | 68.47 | 6.67 |
| Crude protein* | 68.86[a] | 72.46[D] | 5.23 |
| Ether extract | 82.05 | 87.69 | 6.88 |
| Crude fiber* | 53.25[a] | 59.21[D] | 11.20 |
| Nitrogen free extract | 67.37 | 70.47 | 4.61 |
| **Nutritive value (per cent)** | | | |
| CP | 12.48 | 13.29 | 6.49 |
| DCP* | 8.61[a] | 9.65[D] | 12.08 |
| TDN | 64.00 | 68.52 | 7.07 |
| **Milk yield** | | | |
| Milk yield (kg/day) | 4.08 | 4.64 | 13.73 |

* Means bearing different superscripts in a row differ significantly ($P<0.05$).

Naik *et al.,* 2013d.

There are reports of increase in milk yield of 7.8 per cent and 9.3 per cent (FCM yield) (Reddy *et al.,* 1988) and 13.73 per cent (Naik *et al.,* 2013d) due to feeding of hydroponics fodder to lactating cows. The feedback from the farmers of the Satara district of Maharashtra revealed increase in the milk yield by 0.5-2.5 liters per animal per day and net profit by Rs. 25-50/- per animal per day due to feeding of hydroponics fodder to their dairy animals. Besides, the other advantages observed by the farmers were increase in fat and SNF content of the milk, improvement in health and conception rate of the dairy animals, reduction in cattle feed requirement by 25 per cent, increase in taste (sweetness) of the milk, whiter milk, reduction in labour cost, requirement of less space and water, freshness and high palatability of the hydroponics fodder *etc.* (Naik *et al.,* 2013).

## Economics of Production of Hydroponic Fodder

The cost of production of the hydroponics green fodder maize is mainly influenced by the seed, electricity and labour. Seed cost alone contributes about 25 per cent of the total cost of production. It is observed that in the hydroponics green fodder production unit of 600 kg daily production potential, approximately 1500-1600 liters of water (if water is not recycled) and about 15-16 units of electricity are consumed. In the existing condition, the cost of production of the hydroponics green fodder maize is approximately 4.50/kg on fresh basis (Naik *et al.,* 2012b), which is almost similar to the market price of the conventional green fodder. It is worth mentioning here that if the seeds are produced by farmers, the cost of production of the hydroponics fodder will be decreased significantly. To produce about 100 kg hydroponics green fodder maize daily, approximately 6.5 tons maize seeds will be required annually, for which about 0.7-1.0 ha land is required to produce maize seeds depending upon the number of crops per year. Besides, adequate dry fodders (stovers) can also be available for feeding the dairy animals.

During the initial stage, though the cost of fodder produced by hydroponics system and conventional method may the similar; in future, when there will be non-availability of land for production of fodder to the animals, this alternative technology will be able to provide required fodder with very limited land area. Further, with the advancement of time, the cost of machine and its operational cost may go down on a similar manner as has been observed with the mobile phone technology. However, the greatest advantage of hydroponics technology over conventional practices for production of green fodder is that farmer can produce as per the requirement and there is no post-harvest loss.

No doubt, cost of production is the key determinant for the success of any technology, but the most important fact is under which circumstances we are using technology.

## Challenges in Producing Hydroponic Fodder

There are a number of challenges in producing hydroponic fodder. A common challenge that causes many problems for those with fodder sheds is mould. Given the warm moist environment within a fodder shed mould can easily take hold, ruin the crop and cause livestock health issues if fed. Thus, active management of mould risk is essential. Mouldy sprouts have decreased livestock performance in trials (Myers, 1974), and has been known to result in animal deaths.

Mould is actively managed within sheds through pre treatment of the seed. Additives to the water are used for pre-soaking the grain to minimize the risk of mould. Shed hygiene is also important and thus considerable attention is paid to ensuring the growing trays are well cleaned following each crop and prior to the sowing of the new crop.

## Conclusion

Hydroponic fodder production systems produce large quantities of green, palatable livestock feed in limited space/available land. However, the research reviewed and analysis undertaken in this report indicates that there are challenges associated with the production and economic competitiveness of hydroponic fodder relative to alternative feed sources. The costs associated with the establishment and daily operation of a fodder shed, coupled with dry matter yield losses during the sprouting make hydroponic fodder an expensive feed source. This, coupled with a lack of concrete evidence around animal performance on hydroponic fodder will limit the adoption of hydroponic fodder production systems. There is an opportunity for some research to be undertaken to examine the performance of livestock on hydroponic fodder and the attributes of the final product. The production of a product with superior attributes that could generate significant premiums in top level markets may go some way in making hydroponic fodder an economic feed. This would have to be accompanied by a positive production response in the give class of livestock also.

## REFERENCES

Al-Karaki, G.N. and Al-Hashimi, M. (2012). Green fodder production and water use efficiency of some forage crops under hydroponic condition. *Internl. Schol. Res. Network*. DOI: 10.5402/2012/924672.

Anonymous. 2012. Moo-ve aside, hydroponics technology is here. Gomantak Times, 11-10-2012.

Brithal, P.S. and Jha, A.K. (2005). Economic losses due to various constraints in dairy production in India. *Indian Journal of Animal Science*, **75**(12): 1470-1475.

Bull, R. C. and Peterson, C. F. (1969). Nutritive value of sprouted wheat for swine and poultry. *Journal of Animal Science*, (Suppl.), **28**(6): 856

Bustos, C.D.E., Gonzalez, E.L., Aguilera B.A. and Esptnoza, G.J.A. (2000). Forraje Hidropónico, Una Alternativa para la Suplementación Caprina en el Semidesierto Queretano. XXXVIII. Reunión Nacional de Investigación Pecuaria. Puebla, México, 383 pp.

Carruthers, S. (2003). Green Feed – Livestock Fodder Shed. Retrieved from http: //owll.massey.ac.nz/referencing/apa-interactive.php

Chandra, P. and Gupta, M.J. (2003). Cultivation in hi-tech greenhouses for enhanced productivity of natural resources to achive the objective of precision farming. In: Precision Farming in Horticulture (Singh, H.P., Singh, Gorakh, Samuel, J.C. and Pathak, R.K. (Eds). pp. 64-74.

Chavan, J. and Kadam, S.S. (1989). Nutritional improvement of cereals by sprouting. *Critical Reviews of Food Science and Nutrition*, **28**(5): 401-437.

Dikshit, A.K. and Brithal, P.S. (2010). India's livestock feed demand: estimates and projections. *Agricultural Economics Research Review*, **23**: 15-28.

Dung, D.D., Goodwin, I.R. and Nolan, J.V. (2010). Nutrient Content and in sacco digestibility of barley grain and sprouted barley. *Journal of Animal and Veterinary Advances*, **9**(19): 2485-2492.

Fazaeli, H., Golmohammadi, H.A., Shoayee, A.A., Montajebi, N. and Mosharraf, Sh. (2011). Performance of feedlot calves fed hydroponics fodder barley. *Journal of Agricultural Science and Technology*, **13**: 365-375.

Finney, P.L. (1982). Effect of Germination on Cereal and Legume Nutrient Changes and Food or Feed Value: A Comprehensive Review. *Recent Advances In Phytochemistry*, **17**: 229-305.

GoI. (2010). Basic animal husbandry statistics. Department of Animal Husbandry, Dairying and Fisheries, Ministry of Agriculture, Govt. of India, Krishi Bhawan, New Delhi. pp.1-133.

Kohler, G.O., Elvehjem, C.A. and Hart, E.B. (1938). The relation of the grass juice factor to guinea pig nutrition. *The Journal of Nutrition,* **15**(5): 445-459.

Marisco, G., Miscera, E., Dimatteo, S., Minuti, F., Vicenti, A. and Zarrilli, A. (2009). Evaluation of animal welfare and milk production of goat fed on diet containing hydroponically germinating seeds. *Italian Journal of Animal Science,* **8**(2): 625-627.

Mincera, E., Ragni, M., Minuti, F., Rubino, G., Marisco, G. and Zarrilli, A. (2009). Improvement of sheeo welfaee and milk production fed on diet containing hydroponically germinating seeds. *Italian Journal of Animal Science,* **8**(2): 634-636.

Morgan, J., Hunter, R.R. and O'Haire, R. (1992). Limiting factors in hydroponic barley grass production. In: Proc. 8th International Congress on Soilless Culture. Hunter's Rest, South Africa, pp: 241-261.

Mukhopad, Yu. (1994). Cultivating green forage and vegetables in the Buryat Republic. *Mezhdunarodnyi Sel'skokhozyaistvennyi Zhurnal,* **6**: 51-52.

Myers, J. (1974). Feeding Livestock from the Hydroponic Garden. M. Sc. Thesis, Arizona State University.

Naik, P.K., Dhuri, R.B., Karunakaran, M. and Swain, B.K. and Singh, N.P. (2013a). Hydroponics technology for green fodder production. Indian Dairyman, **65**: 54-58.

Naik, P.K., Dhuri, R.B. and Singh, N.P. (2011). Technology for production and feeding of hydroponics green fodder. Extension Folder No. 45/2011, ICAR Research Complex for Goa, Goa.

Naik, P.K., Dhuri, R.B., Swain, B.K. and Singh, N.P. (2012a). Nutrient changes with the growth of hydroponics fodder maize. *Indian Journal of Animal Nutrition,* **29**: 161-163.

Naik, P.K., Dhuri, R.B., Swain, B.K. and Singh, N.P. (2012b). Cost of production of hydroponics fodder maize. In: Proc. of 8th Biennial Animal Nutrition Association Conference on 'Animal Nutrition Research Strategies for Food Security', November 28-30, 2012, Bikaner, Rajasthan, India, p.12.

Naik, P.K., Dhuri, R.B., Swain, B.K. and Singh, N.P. (2013c). Water management for green fodder production as livestock feed in Goa. In: Abstracts of International Conference on 'Water Management for Climate Resilient Agriculture' held at Jalgaon, Maharashtra, India, May 28-31, 2012, pp. 126-127.

Naik, P.K., Dhuri, R.B., Swain, B.K., Karunakaran, M. and Singh, N.P. 2013d. Effect of feeding hydroponics maize fodder on digestibility of nutrients and milk production in lactating cows. In: Proceedings of National Conference on 'Current Nutritional Concepts for Productivity Enhancement in Livestock and Poultry' held at Madras Veterinary College, Chennai, Tamilnadu, India, August 29-30, 2013, pp. 98-99.

Naik, P.K., Gaikwad, S.P., Gupta, M.J., Dhuri, R.B., Dhumal, G.M. and Singh, N.P. (2013b). Low cost devices for hydroponics fodder production. *Indian Dairyman*, **65**: 68-72.

Naik, P.K. (2012). Hydroponics technology for fodder production. ICAR News, **18**(3): 4.

Naik, P.K. and Singh, N.P. (2013). Hydroponics fodder production: an alternative technology for sustainable livestock production against impeding climate change. In: compendium of Model Training Course 'Management Strategies for Sustainable Livestock Production against Impending Climate Change', held during November 18-25, 2013. Southern Regional Station, National Dairy Research Institute, Adugodi, Bengaluru, India, pp. 70-75.

Naik, P.K. and Singh, N.P. (2014). Production and feeding of hydroponics green fodder. *Indian Farming*, **64**(6): 42-44.

Pandey, H.N. and Pathak, N.N. (1991). Nutritional evaluation of artificially grown barley fodder in lactating crossbred cows. *Indian Journal of Animal Nutrition*, **8**(1): 77-78.

Rajendra, P., Seghal, J.P., Patnayak, B.C. and Beniwal, R.K. (1998). Utilization of artificially grown barley fodder by sheep. *Indian Journal of Small Ruminant*, **4**(2): 63-68.

Reddy, G.V.N., Reddy, M.R. and Reddy, K.K. (1988). Nutrient utilization by milch cattle fed on rations containing artificially grown fodder. *Indian Journal of Animal Nutrition*, **5**(1): 19-22.

Resh, H.M. (2001). Hydroponic Food Production, 6$^{th}$ ed., 567 pp., Woodbridge Press, Santa Barbara, CA.

Rodriguez-Muela, C., Rodriguez, H.E., Ruiz, O., Flores, A., Grado, J.A. and Arzola, C. (2004). Use of green fodder produced in hydroponic system as supplement for lactating cows during the dry season. In the *Proceeding of the American Society of Animal Science*, pp. 271-274.

Sneath, R. and Mclntosh, F. (2003). Review of hydroponic fodder production for beef cattle. Queensland Government Department of Primary Industries, Dalby, Queensland.

Snow, A.M., Ghaly, A.E. and Snow, A. (2008). A comparative assessment of hydroponically grown cereal crops for the purification of aquaculture waste water and the production of fish feed. *American Journal of Agricultural Biology Science,* **3**(1): 364-378.

Tudor, G., Darcy, T., Smith, P. and Shallcross, F. (2003). The intake and live weight change of drought master steers fed hydroponically grown young sprouted barley fodder (Autograss), Department of Agriculture, Western Australia.

## Chapter 22

# Quantification of Pesticide Residues in Advanced Analytical Method

*R.P. Singh*

*Nanaji Deshmukh Veterinary Science University,*
*Jabalpur, Madhya Pradesh*

With increasing consumer awareness and stringent regulatory guidelines there is an urgent need for monitoring and control of pesticide residues entering the food chain. Under the current intensive production mode, the usages of pesticides in crop protection, food storage and as ectoparasiticides in veterinary are inevitable. Presently, about 1000 active ingredients have been registered that can be grouped into more than 40 classes of chemical families. The levels of pesticides in feed and foods of animal origin have become a relevant issue in this food safety era.

Pesticides exposure can be measured through the biomonitoring of either the parent compounds or their metabolites in body fluids and tissues. Chromatography remains workhorse technique for pesticides estimation even today. The High Performance Liquid Chromatography (HPLC) methods for quantification of polar pesticides are viable and cheaper way of bio-monitoring, in order to reduce the incidence of violative residues in feeds of animals and foods of animal origin destined for human consumption.

**Pesticide:** Cypermethrin

## Standard/Working Solutions

- ☆ Stock solution of Cypermethrin 1 mg/ml in acetonitrile
- ☆ Working standard solution 1, 0.5, 0.25 pg/ml in acetonitrile

## Equipments

1. Ultrasonicator
2. Filtration unit assembly
3. Membrane filter: Solvent filter (0.2 pm) and Syringe filter (0.2 pm)
4. Blender (Homogenizer)
5. Vortexer
6. Referigerated centrifuge
7. The HPLC system consisted of Quaternary gradient pump and detector.
8. HPLC column (Phenomex) Cis 4-6 x 250 mm x 4 pm particle size

## Stepwise Sample Extraction Procedure

- Cut 100 g of meat into small pieces (2-3 mm) and blend it for 2 min by using a blender.
- Take 10 g of this blended meat and homogenize it in 10 ml of Mill-Q water.
- Add 2 ml of acetonitrile to 0.5 g of the homogenate, and vortex it for 1.5 min to mix well and keep the mixture undisturbed for 10 min.
- To this add 1 ml HPLC grade water and vortex again for 1 min.
- Centrifuge at 3000 rpm for 20 min in a refrigerated centrifuge.
- Collect 0.5 ml of the supernatant and add 0.5 ml of HPLC grade water in a separate test tube.
- Vortex for 1 min and centrifuge at 10,000 rpm for 10 min.
- Collect the resultant supernatant and filter by using 0.22 (xm nylon filter.
- Inject 20 |xl of this aliquot into HPLC system.

## HPLC Assay Conditions

| | | |
|---|---|---|
| Column | : | $C_{18}$ 4.6 x 250 mm x 4µm particle size, |
| Mobile Phase (Isocratic elution) | : | HPLC water: Acetonitrile (40: 60, v/v) |
| Wavelength | : | 220 nm |
| Flow-rate | : | 0.6 ml/min |
| Column temperature | : | 40°C |

## Quantification of Cypermethrin

- The quantification of cypermethrin in test sample is done by comparing with working standard solution.
- Cypermethrin concentration is calculated as follows: Cypermethrin (ppb)= [$A_t$ x Cs x PF x DF]/As

*where,*

$A_1$ = Area of test sample,

As = Area of standard sample,

$C_s$ = Concentration of standard solution, PF= Purity factor,

DF= Dilution factor

## REFERENCES

FAO/WHO Standards 2011. Pesticides residues in food. Maximum residues limits. CODEX Alimentarius. http: //www.codexalimentarius. net/mrls/pestdes/ jsp/pest_q- e.jsp

Rodriguez-Cuesta, M.J., Boque, R., Rius, F.X., Martinez Vidal, J.L. and Garrido Frenich, A. 2005. *Chemomelrics and Intelligent Laboratory Systems,* 77: 251.

Zhi, M.L., Xiao, H.Z., Wei, H.L., Chun, W. and Zhi, W. 2009. *Chinese Chemical Letters,* 20: 213-216.

## Chapter 23

# Estimation of Heavy Metals in Biological Samples Using Atomic Absorption Spectrophotometry

*Ankur Khare, Sunil Nayak, R.P.S. Baghel and Nagendra Uikey*

*Department of Animal Nutrition, College of Veterinary Science and Animal Husbandry, Nanaji Deshmukh Veterinary Science University, Jabalpur, Madhya Pradesh*

Heavy metals are widespread pollutants of environment. Bioaccumulation of heavy metals in the food chain imposes a potential risk to animal and human health. Research studies on the effects of heavy metal exposure on health and performance of animals largely depends on the accurate determination of heavy metal concentration in the biological sample. For the estimation of heavy metals in the biological samples Atomic Absorption Spectrophotometry is one of the most accurate analytical techniques. The phenomenon of atomic absorption pertains to the absorption of radiant energy by free atoms in their ground state.

The technique makes use of the wavelengths of light specifically absorbed by an element. Substances when dispersed in the form of atomic vapor (flame) are able to absorb their characteristic radiations identical to those which the same substance can emit. It is this property, which forms the basis of Atomic Absorption Spectrophoto- metry. An atomic absorption spectrophotometer consists of a light source, a sample compartment and a detector. In this method, light from a source is directed through the sample to detector. The source of light is a lamp whose cathode is composed of the element being measured. Each element requires a different lamp. A suitable quantity of the sample material is oxidized (wet digestion) with a mixture of acids and brought into solution with triple-distilled water. The acid digested solution is then used for the estimation of heavy metals.

## Wet Oxidation (Digestion) of the Samples

In wet oxidation (digestion), minerals are solubilised without volatilization. The wet digestion of samples is carried out by triple m id (perchloric, sulphuric and nitric acids in the ratio of 0.5:1:4) digestion method A brief description of the procedure for wet oxidation of feeds/fodder mid blood sample is given below:

### Reagents and Glass Wares

Sulphuric acid, Nitric acid and Perchloric acid of A.R. Grades, triple glass distilled water, Pyrex/Corning glass wares.

### Procedure

Feeds/fodder samples: Weigh accurately 1-2 g fresh sample and transfer it into a 100 ml Kjeldahl flask. Add 2 ml water and 2 ml of sulpluric n acid and 2 glass beads. Heat the mixture gently over an electrical micro-digestion bench till a homogenous dark brown liquid is formed. After cooling the flask, add 0.5 ml perchloric acid and 5.0 ml nitric acid and heat again till the dark brown colour becomes faint. Cool the flask again, add 2.5 ml nitric acid and heat again till the material changes to light yellow or colourless mass. At this stage, add 5 drops of perchloric acid (after removing from the heaters) to ensure the removal of even the traces of organic matter. Heat again until thick white fumes of perchloric acid no longer comes out. Add little water to the flask, while still warm, to keep the solid salts (formed in the final stages of digestion) in solution state. Make a suitable volume of the digested sample in a volumetric flask with triple glass-distilled water for further analysis in AAS. If required the sample may be filtered.

### Blood

Take 5 ml blood in a test tube. Add 1 ml sulphuric acid and 2 glass beads. Heat the tubes continuously over an electrical micro-digestion bench, until the dark brown liquid is formed. Cool the tubes, add 0.5 ml perchloric acid and 2.5 ml of nitric acid. Resume heating till it becomes light yellow or colourless. At this stage add 5 drops of perchloric acid and heat again till white fumes of perchloric acid no longer appear. A little distilled water is added to the tubes, while warm to keep the solid salts in solution.

## Estimation by Atomic Absorption Spectrophotometry

A PC based Double beam Atomic Absorption Spectrophotometer suitable for absorption and emission analysis having Back-ground Correction and Flame Emission capability will be used for quantitative elemental analysis by measuring the absorbance of a sample atomized in a flame. The test material (acid digest) in solution is delivered through nebuliser (reduced to a spray) into a spray chamber as a mist, wherein it is mixed with the entering stream of oxidizer and fuel gases (air/acetylene or air/nitrous oxide) and passed through the burner where it is atomized (*i.e.*m the material is dissociated into free atoms) in the flame (2500°C air/acetylene and 3000-3500°C air/nitrous oxide). Generally oxyacetylene flame is used, which is obtained by supplying dry and dust-free air through a compressor and acetylene through a gas cylinder.

The source of radiation used is a hollow cathode lamp as described earlier. The modulated light from the Hollow Cathode lamp splits into two beams, a Sample and a Reference beam. The Sample beam travels through the flame while the Reference beam travels around it. The reference signal is used to compensate for the drifts in lamp intensities. The sample signal is processed for photometric computations (per cent T, ABS or Cone.) by PC.

Quantitative analysis can be achieved by measuring the absorbance of a series of solutions of known concentration (standard solutions). A calibration curve and the equation for the line can be used to determine an unknown concentration based on its absorbance. As with other spectrophotometric techniques the Beer-Lambert law is applicable to AAS also. Accordingly the absorbance is proportional to the concentration of atoms in the flame and in turn the concentration of the element in the measured solution.

Instrument parameters and calibration parameters can be stored as Applications, which can be retrieved as and when required. Standard conditions for the estimation of cadmium, mercury, lead by atomic absorption spectrophotmetry are given below:

| *Standard Conditions* | *Metal* | | |
|---|---|---|---|
| | *Cadmium (Cd)* | *Mercury (Hg)* | *Lead (Pb)* |
| Wavelength | 228.8 nm | 253.6 nm | 217.0 |
| Slit setting | 0.5 nm | 0.5 nm | 1.0 nm |
| Operating current | 5 mA | 5 mA | 5 mA |
| Sensitivity | 0.04 μg/ml | 3.0μg/ml (Upto 0.001μg/ml using VGA) | 0.25 μg/ml |

Hollow cathode lamp of respective element as light source and Air-acetylene flame type is used in all the analysis.

## REFERENCES

Garg, A.K. and Shyam Karan. 2014. Heavy Metal Estimation in Meat Sample. In: *Nutrition, Productivity and Product Quality in Farm Animals,* (Eds. Jadhav, S.E., Pattanaik, A.K., Dutta, N., Garg, A.K. and Verma, A.K), Indian Veterinary Research Institute, Izatnagar, India, pp. 183-183.

## Chapter 24

# Estimation of Short Chain Fatty Acids and Methane by Gas Liquid Chromatography

*Ankur Khare, Sunil Nayak, R.P.S. Baghel and Pramod Sharma*

*Department of Animal Nutrition, College of Veterinary Science and Animal Husbandry, Nanaji Deshmukh Veterinary Science University, Jabalpur, Madhya Pradesh*

Gas Liquid Chromtography (GLC) is a very quick, efficient and precise method for the analysis of various small chain fatty acids and methane. The chromatography system is termed as GLC because here stationary phase is a liquid and mobile phase is a gas. It works on the principle of partition chromatography. The ratio of the concentration of a solute in two phases is called its partition coefficient. The whole unit of GLC includes:

- *Injector*: For loading of sample on the column
- *Column*: Tubing (glass or stainless steel) packed with stationary phase
- *Detector*: For measuring the quantity of separated components
- *Oven and Heaters*: For temperature control of column, detector and injector
- *Carrier gas*: To provide a suitable gas flow through the column this can take with them the components of the mixture. The commonly used carrier gases are nitrogen, hydrogen, argon and helium

A sample is injected into the column along with carrier gas near the head of packed chromatographic column. Separation of various components of the sample occurs as a result of multiple forces by which the column material tends to retain these components. All components pass through the column at varying speeds and emerge in the inverse order of their retention by the column material. Upon emerging from the column, the gaseous phase immediately enters a detector attached to the column. Here the individual components register a series of signals which appear as peaks on the chromatogram. The chromatographic peaks are used for qualitative and quantitative detection of the components.

## Conditions for Fractionation of Volatile Fatty Acids on GLC

A mixture of volatile fatty acids can be fractionated on GLC, by using following conditions:

- ✰ The detector is Flame Ionization Detector (F.I.D.).
- ✰ Column is packed with cromosorb 101 and the size of the column is 1/8 diameter and 4 feet length
- ✰ Flow rate: Nitrogen, 30 ml/min (carrier gas); hydrogen, 30 ml/min and air 320 ml/min
- ✰ Temperature: Injector, 240°C; column oven, 172°C and detector, 240°C.
- ✰ Sample size: 1μl

## Preparation of Sample

Draw rumen liquor from a cannulated animal and filter it through 4 layers of muslin cloth. Take 5 ml of strained rumen liquor, add to 1ml metaphosphoric acid (25 per cent). Metaphosphoric acid precipitates the proteins which otherwise contaminate the column. Stand the sample for 30 min and then centrifuge it at 5000 rpm for 10 min. Process the sample at 4°C. Collect the clear supernatant and use for analysis.

**Table 24.1. Working Standard Mixture of Acids (10 ml)**

| *Acid* | *Acid Mix (ml/10 ml)* | *Final Concentration (mg/ml)* | *mM/100 ml* |
|---|---|---|---|
| Acitic acid | 1.68 | 4.2 | 7.00 |
| Propionic acid | 0.48 | 1.2 | 1.62 |
| Isobutyric acid | 0.12 | 0.3 | 0.34 |
| Butyric acid | 0.24 | 0.6 | 0.68 |
| Isovaleric acid | 0.12 | 0.3 | 0.29 |
| Valeric acid | 0.12 | 0.3 | 0.29 |
| Distilled water | Make the volume to 10 ml | | |

## Preparation of Standard

Stock solution of acid: Take 250 mg acetic acid in a volumetric flusk and make it to 10 ml with distilled water. The concentration of the solution is 25mg/ml. Likewise prepare stock solution of each acid.

## Procedure

Switch on gas chromatograph sequentially in the following manner:

- ☆ Make repeat 1.0μl injections using 10 (xl Hamilton liquid syringe of the composite working standard until a stable response is obtained. Under these conditions, the analysis of rumen liquor takes about 8 min from acetic to valeric acid.
- ☆ Now inject 1μl of sample and have chromatogram of the sample.

## Calculations

Calculate mM/100 ml of each acid in the strained rumen liquor from the expression:

Peak area = Height of the peak x half of the peak width

$$\text{Cone, of unknown} = \frac{\text{Peak area of sample x standard conc. x df}}{\text{Peak area of standard}}$$

Where, df = Dilution factor

### *Note*

Supply of carrier gas to the instrument should be stopped only when the column and detector temperature has fallen to near ambient temperature. Column should **not** be allowed to remain in a heated oven without a flow of carrier gas, it will spoil the column.

## Estimation of Methane by GLC

### Conditions for Methane Estimation

- ☆ Detector: Flame Ionization Detector (F.I.D.).
- ☆ Column: Porapak-Q column
- ☆ Gas flow rate: Nitrogen, 20 ml/min; hydrogen, 30 ml/min and air 300 ml/min
- ☆ Temperature: Injector 50°C, column oven 40°C and detector 50°C
- ☆ Sample size: 100μl

### Standard

The standard gas for methane estimation consists of 50 per cent methane and 50 per cent carbon dioxide. Of this mixture 25μl is injected in the column *i.e.*, 12.5μl of methane. The volume of the standard can be changed according to the expected concentration of unknown sample.

## Sample

The gas produced in the fermentation vessel can be directly used for methane estimation. With the help of Hamilton gas tight syringe, inject 100µl gas. Care should be taken that no water traces should enter the column. The concentration can be calculated as mentioned for VFA.

## Chapter 25

# Establish of Rumen Microbiology Laboratory and Identification of Microbes

*Anju Nayak, Joycee Jogi, Vandana Gupta, Ajay Rai and Smita Bordoloi*

*Department of Veterinary Microbiology, College of Veterinary Science and Animal Husbandry, Nanaji Deshmukh Veterinary Science University, Jabalpur, Madhya Pradesh*

## Essential Equipment for Rumen Microbiology Laboratory

1. Thermo-cycler
2. Spectrophotometer
3. Gas chromatograph
4. High performance liquid chromatograph
5. Microscope: Compound and Phase contrast
6. Autoclave
7. Hot air oven
8. Shaking Incubator
9. Anaerobic work station
10. Water bath
11. pH meter

12. Magnetic stirrer
13. Vortex mixer
14. Weighing balance
15. Freeze dryer
16. High speed refrigerated
17. Micro centrifuge refrigerated
18. Electrophoresis equipment
19. Gas cylinder for hydrogen, nitrogen and carbon dioxide Grade-1
20. Gas purification apparatus (for removal of oxygen)

## Working in Microbiology Laboratory

1. Working in a microbiology laboratory may expose the researchers to many hazards like strong acids, alkalis, toxic compounds carcinogens, pathogenic microbes, high voltage, radiations *etc.* But exposure to pathogens is the most dangerous as it not only affects the researcher,but he/she also carries infection to his/her families or friends and may act as a carrier of the pathogen.

   Fortunately most of the rumen microbes are non –pathogenic. But while working with animals, one may get exposure to microbes of zoonotic importance. Therefore precautions essential for a clinical microbiology laboratory are also applicable to a rumen microbiology laboratory.
2. Oral pipetting should always be avoided.
3. Care should be taken that no drop of culture falls from the used pipette. These drops may form aerosol, which may be a source of infection.
4. Cotton plugs, screw caps, rubber and aluminums caps, pipettes, pipette tips, and other used material should be disposed off properly in a disinfective solution.
5. Centrifugation of a microbial culture of a liquid containing live microbes should be done very carefully as it is one of the most potent sources of infection.
6. Extra care should be taken while autoclaving. After autoclaving, open the autoclave chamber lid after cooling it.

## Precautions

1. Make it a habit to wash your hands with anti-septic soap immediately on entering and before leaving the laboratory, even if you are sure you did not touch any microbial culture during your stay in the laboratory.
2. Always wear a laboratory apron, which must be clean and washed and rinsed with anti-septic solution frequently.

3. The working space should be kept clean and microbes free. Rinse the place with anti-septic solution before and after completion of the work.
4. While working in the laboratory never bring your hands near the mouth.
5. Never keep drinking water or eatables in the same fridge in which microbial cultures or chemicals are stored.
6. Avoid eating anything in the laboratory.
7. All the glassware and plastic ware should be sterilized before washing or disposing it off.
8. While working with biological material like rumen liquor, rumen content, faeces, serum or other biological fluids, care must be taken to avoid contact with the skin and accidental spilling over the body parts or eyes.

## Identification of Microbes

To study the morphology of bacteria its fixation and staining is essential. There are different methods of staining as mentioned below:

### Simple Staining

Simple staining includes one stain for visualization of only shape and size of microbes since it imparts same colour to all types of bacteria. Dyes used are Aqueous Methylene Blue, Loffler's Alkaline Methylene Blue and Carbol Fuchsin.

### Aqueous Methylene Blue

This is a simple bacterial stain for routine use. This stain is also used for acid fast staining as counter stain in Ziehl- Neelsen's method.

#### Materials

Methylene blue stain and *E.coli* culture plate.

#### Method

1. Flame a clean slide, holding it by one corner.
2. Place one loopful of normal saline on the center of the slide with the help of inoculation loop.
3. With a sterilized inoculation loop touch the growth on slant agar lightly and transfer a very little of the colony to the drop and spread in a circular motion.
4. Flame the inoculation loop and allow it to cool.
5. Allow the smear to dry in air.
6. Pour the stain and allow it to act for one minute.
7. Wash the slide with running water and examine the slide under the microscope, using oil immersion.

## Negetive Staining

Instead of staining bacteria only their background is stained. The organism are seen as clear transparent object in a stained background. The commonly used stains are Nigrosin and Indian Ink.

### Materials Required

Clean slides, cover glasses, Inoculation loop, Bunsen burner, Nigrosin solution, *E. coli* culture, Canada balsam and Microscope.

### Method

1. Flame a clean slide, holding it by one corner.
2. Place one loopful of stain on the center of the slide.
3. Touch the growth on slant agar lightly with a sterilized inoculation loop and transfer a very little of the material to the drop and mix it properly.
4. Flame the inoculation loop and allow it to cool.
5. Allow the mixture to dry in air.
6. Examine the slide under the microscope, using oil immersion.
7. Select suitable field under the microscope, draw it.

## Gram's Staining

The most widely used staining procedure in microbiology is the Gram stain, discovered by the Danish scientist and physician Hans Christian Joachim Gram in 1884. It differentiates all bacteria into 2 groups

Gram positive bacteria show violet/blue colour while negative pink colour.

### Materials

Crystal violet stain, Gram's iodine, Ehtyl alcohol (decolourizer), Safranin counter stain and young culture plates of *E. coli* and *Staphylococcus* spp.

### Method

1. Prepare a thin bacterial smear in normal saline, dry in air and fix by passing through the flame.
2. Flood the slide with Crystal violet stain and allow staining for one minute.
3. Wash the slide with running tap water.
4. Add Gram's iodine solution and allow acting for 30 seconds.
5 Wash the slide with tap water and blot dry.
6. Flood the slide with decolourser gently agitating the slide for 30seconds till no more colour comes out from the smear. Blot dry.
7. Counter stain the slide for 20-30 seconds with safranin solution.

8. Wash the slide with tap water and air dry it.
9. Examine the slide under the microscope, using oil immersion.
10. Select suitable field under the microscope, draw it.

# Index

## P



## R



## S



## T



## U



## V



## W